Volume IX
Report No. 91
November 1974

The Community Worker: A Response to Human Need

Formulated by the
Committee on Therapeutic Care

Group for the Advancement of Psychiatry

This publication was produced for the Group for the Advancement of Psychiatry by the Mental Health Materials Center, Inc., New York.

Additional copies of this GAP Publication No. 91 are available at the following prices: 1-9 copies, $3.50 each; 10-24 copies, list less 15 per cent; 25-99 copies, list less 20 per cent; 100-499 copies, list less 30 per cent.

Upon request the Publications Office of the Group for the Advancement of Psychiatry will provide a complete listing of GAP titles currently in print, quantity prices, and information on subscriptions assuring the receipt of new publications as they are released.

Orders amounting to less than $5.00 must be accompanied by remittance. All prices are subject to change without notice.

Please send your order and remittance to: Publications Office, Group for the Advancement of Psychiatry, 419 Park Avenue South, New York, New York 10016.

International Standard Book Number 087318-128-x

Library of Congress Catalog Card Number 62-2872

Printed in the United States of America

TABLE OF CONTENTS

This is the first in a series of publications comprising Volume IX. For a list of other GAP publications on current topics of interest, please see last page of book herein.

STATEMENT OF PURPOSE

The Group for the Advancement of Psychiatry has a membership of approximately 300 psychiatrists, most of whom are organized in the form of a number of working committees. These committees direct their efforts toward the study of various aspects of psychiatry and the application of this knowledge to the fields of mental health and human relations.

Collaboration with specialists in other disciplines has been and is one of GAP's working principles. Since the formation of GAP in 1946 its members have worked closely with such other specialists as anthropologists, biologists, economists, statisticians, educators, lawyers, nurses, psychologists, sociologists, social workers, and experts in mass communication, philosophy, and semantics. GAP envisages a continuing program of work according to the following aims:

1. To collect and appraise significant data in the fields of psychiatry, mental health, and human relations
2. To reevaluate old concepts and to develop and test new ones
3. To apply the knowledge thus obtained for the promotion of mental health and good human relations

GAP is an independent group, and its reports represent the composite findings and opinions of its members only, guided by its many consultants.

THE COMMUNITY WORKER: A RESPONSE TO HUMAN NEED *was formulated by the Committee on Therapeutic Care which acknowledges on page 9 the participation of former Committee members in preparation of this report. The current members of this committee, as well as other committees and the officers of the GAP, are listed below.*

Committee on Therapeutic Care
Robert W. Gibson, Towson, Md., Chr.
Bernard Bandler, Boston
Thomas E. Curtis, Chapel Hill
Harold A. Greenberg, Silver Spring, Md.
Milton Kramer, Cincinnati
Orlando B. Lightfoot, Boston
Melvin Sabshin, Chicago
Benjamin Simon, Boston
Robert E. Switzer, Topeka

Committee on Adolescence
Joseph D. Noshpitz, Washington, Chr.
Maurice R. Friend, New York
Warren J. Gadpaille, Englewood, Colo.
Charles A. Malone, Philadelphia
Silvio J. Onesti, Jr., Belmont, Mass.
Jeanne Spurlock, Silver Spring, Md.
Sidney L. Werkman, Denver

Committee on Aging
Prescott W. Thompson, San Jose, Chr.
Robert N. Butler, Washington, D. C.
Charles M. Gaitz, Houston
Alvin I. Goldfarb, New York
Lawrence F. Greenleigh, Los Angeles
Maurice E. Linden, Philadelphia
Robert D. Patterson, Lexington, Mass.
F. Conyers Thompson, Jr., Atlanta
Montague Ullman, Ardsley, N.Y.
Jack Weinberg, Chicago

Committee on Child Psychiatry
Joseph M. Green, Tucson, Ariz., Chr.
Paul L. Adams, Miami
E. James Anthony, St. Louis
James M. Bell, Canaan, N.Y.
Harlow Donald Dunton, New York
Joseph Fischoff, Detroit
John F. Kenward, Chicago
Ake Mattsson, Charlottesville
John F. McDermott, Jr., Honolulu
Theodore Shapiro, New York
Exie E. Welsch, New York
Virginia N. Wilking, New York

Committee on the College Student
Robert L. Arnstein, Hamden, Conn., Chr.
Harrison P. Eddy, New York
Malkah Tolpin Notman, Brookline, Mass.
Gloria C. Onque, Pittsburgh
Kent E. Robinson, Towson, Md.
Earle Silber, Chevy Chase, Md.
Tom G. Stauffer, White Plains, N.Y.

Committee on the Family
Joseph Satten, San Francisco, Chr.
C. Christian Beels, Bronx, N.Y.
Ivan Boszormenyi-Nagy, Wyncote, Pa.
Murray Bowen, Chevy Chase
Henry U. Grunebaum, Boston
Margaret M. Lawrence, Pomona, N.Y.
David Mendell, Houston
Carol Nadelson, Boston
Norman L. Paul, Cambridge
Israel Zwerling, Philadelphia

Committee on Governmental Agencies
Paul Chodoff, Washington, D.C., Chr.
William S. Allerton, Richmond
Albert M. Biele, Philadelphia
Sidney S. Goldensohn, Jamaica, N.Y.
John E. Nardini, Washington, D.C.
Donald B. Peterson, Fulton, Mo.
Harvey L. P. Resnik, Chevy Chase, Md.
Harold Rosen, Baltimore
Harvey Lee Ruben, New Haven

Committee on International Relations
Bryant M. Wedge, Washington, D.C., Chr.
Francis F. Barnes, Chevy Chase
Eric A. Baum, Cambridge
Alexander Gralnick, Port Chester, N.Y.
Rita R. Rogers, Torrance, Calif.
Bertram H. Schaffner, New York
Mottram P. Torre, New Orleans
Roy M. Whitman, Cincinnati
Ronald M. Wintrob, Hartford

Committee on Medical Education
Saul I. Harrison, Ann Arbor, Chr.
Raymond Feldman, Boulder, Colo.
David R. Hawkins, Charlottesville
Harold I. Lief, Philadelphia
John E. Mack, Chestnut Hill, Mass.
Robert Alan Senescu, New York
Bryce Templeton, Philadelphia
Paul Tyler Wilson, Bethesda, Md.

Committee on Mental Health Services
W. Walter Menninger, Topeka, Chr.
Allan Beigel, Tucson, Ariz.
Eugene M. Caffey, Jr., Washington, D.C.
Merrill T. Eaton, Omaha
James B. Funkhouser, Richmond, Va.
Robert S. Garber, Belle Mead, N.J.
Stanley Hammons, Frankfort, Ky.
Donald Scherl, Boston
Jack A. Wolford, Pittsburgh

Committee on Mental Retardation
Henry H. Work, Washington, D.C., Chr.
Howard V. Bair, Parsons, Kans.
Norman R. Bernstein, Boston

Andrew P. Morrison, Cambridge
William C. Offenkrantz, Chicago
William L. Peltz, Manchester, Vt.
Franz K. Reichsman, Brooklyn
Lewis L. Robbins, Glen Oaks, N.Y.
Richard I. Shader, Newton Centre, Mass.
Harley C. Shands, New York
Joseph P. Tupin, Sacramento
Herbert Weiner, Bronx, N.Y.

CONTRIBUTING MEMBERS
Carlos C. Alden, Jr., Buffalo
Charlotte G. Babcock, Pittsburgh
Grace Baker, New York
Walter E. Barton, Washington, D. C.
Spencer Bayles, Houston, Tex.
Anne R. Benjamin, Chicago
Ivan C. Berlien, Coral Gables, Fla.
Sidney Berman, Washington, D. C.
Grete L. Bibring, Cambridge
Edward G. Billings, Denver
Carl A. L. Binger, Cambridge
H. Waldo Bird, St. Louis
Wilfred Bloomberg, Boston
H. Keith H. Brodie, Baltimore
Eugene Brody, Menlo Park, Calif.
Matthew Brody, Brooklyn, N.Y.
Ewald W. Busse, Durham
Dale Cameron, Guilford, Conn.
Gerald Caplan, Boston
Hugh T. Carmichael, Washington, D. C.
Ian L. W. Clancey, Maitland, Ont., Can.
Sanford I. Cohen, Boston
Jules V. Coleman, New Haven
Robert Coles, Cambridge
Frank J. Curran, New York
William D. Davidson, Washington, D. C.
Leonard J. Duhl, Berkeley
Lloyd C. Elam, Nashville
Joel Elkes, Baltimore
Joseph T. English, New York
Louis C. English, Pomona, N.Y.
O. Spurgeon English, Narberth, Pa.
Dana L. Farnsworth, Boston
Stuart M. Finch, Tucson, Ariz.
Alfred Flarsheim, Chicago
Archie R. Foley, New York
Alan Frank, Albuquerque, N. M.
Daniel X. Freedman, Chicago
Albert J. Glass, Chicago
Louis A. Gottschalk, Irvine, Calif.
Milton Greenblatt, Sepulveda, Calif.
Maurice H. Greenhill, Scarsdale, N. Y.
John H. Greist, Indianapolis
Roy R. Grinker, Sr., Chicago
Ernest M. Gruenberg, Poughkeepsie, N. Y.
Edward O. Harper, Cleveland, Ohio
Mary O'Neill Hawkins, New York
J. Cotter Hirschberg, Topeka
Edward J. Hornick, New York
Joseph Hughes, Philadelphia
Portia Bell Hume, Berkeley
Irene M. Josselyn, Phoenix
Jay Katz, New Haven
Sheppard G. Kellam, Chicago
Marion E. Kenworthy, New York
Gerald L. Klerman, Boston
Othilda M. Krug, Cincinnati
Zigmond M. Lebensohn, Washington, D. C.
Henry D. Lederer, Washington, D. C.
Robert L. Leopold, Philadelphia
Alan I. Levenson, Tucson, Ariz.
Earl A. Loomis, New York
Reginald S. Lourie, Washington, D. C.
Alfred O. Ludwig, Boston
Jeptha R. MacFarlane, Westbury, N. Y.
Sidney G. Margolin, Denver
Helen V. McLean, Chicago
John A. MacLeod, Cincinnati
Jack H. Mendelson, Belmont, Mass.
Karl A. Menninger, Topeka
James G. Miller, Louisville, Ky.
John A. P. Millet, Nyack, N. Y.
Peter B. Neubauer, New York
Rudolph G. Novick, Lincolnwood, Ill.
Lucy D. Ozarin, Bethesda, Md.
Irving Philips, San Francisco
Charles A. Pinderhughes, Boston
Eveoleen N. Rexford, Cambridge
Milton Rosenbaum, Bronx, N. Y.
W. Donald Ross, Cincinnati
Lester H. Rudy, Chicago
David S. Sanders, Beverly Hills
Kurt O. Schlesinger, San Francisco
Elvin V. Semrad, Boston
Calvin F. Settlage, Sausalito, Calif.
Benson R. Snyder, Cambridge
John P. Spiegel, Waltham, Mass.
Brandt F. Steele, Denver
Eleanor A. Steele, Denver
Rutherford B. Stevens, New York
Alan A. Stone, Cambridge, Mass.
Perry C. Talkington, Dallas
Graham C. Taylor, Montreal

Lloyd J. Thompson, Chapel Hill
Harvey J. Tompkins, New York
Lucia E. Tower, Chicago
Arthur F. Valenstein, Cambridge
Suzanne T. van Amerongen, Boston
Harold M. Visotsky, Chicago
Robert S. Wallerstein, San Francisco
Andrew S. Watson, Ann Arbor
Edward M. Weinshel, San Francisco
Joseph B. Wheelwright, San Francisco
Robert L. Williams, Houston
David G. Wright, Providence
Stanley F. Yolles, Stony Brook, N. Y.

LIFE MEMBERS
S. Spafford Ackerly, Louisville
Kenneth E. Appel, Ardmore, Pa.
Malcolm J. Farrell, Waverley, Mass.
William S. Langford, New York
Benjamin Simon, Boston
Francis H. Sleeper, Augusta, Me.

LIFE CONSULTANT
Mrs. Ethel L. Ginsburg, New York

BOARD OF DIRECTORS

OFFICERS

President
Judd Marmor, M.D.
2025 Zonal Avenue
Los Angeles, Calif. 90033

Vice President
John C. Nemiah, M.D.
330 Brookline Avenue
Boston, Mass. 02215

Secretary
Jack A. Wolford, M.D.
3811 O'Hara Street
Pittsburgh, Pa. 15213

Treasurer
Gene L. Usdin, M.D.
1522 Aline Street
New Orleans, La. 70115

Immediate Past President
George Tarjan, M.D.
700 Westwood Plaza
Los Angeles, Calif. 90024

Board Members
C. Knight Aldrich
Viola W. Bernard
Robert N. Butler
Leo Madow
Charles B. Wilkinson

Honorary Member
Malcolm J. Farrell

Past Presidents, ex-Officio

Jack R. Ewalt	1951-53
Walter E. Barton	1953-55
Dana L. Farnsworth	1957-59
Marion E. Kenworthy	1959-61
Henry W. Brosin	1961-63
Leo H. Bartemeier	1963-65
Robert S. Garber	1965-67
Herbert C. Modlin	1967-69
John Donnelly	1969-71

Deceased Past Presidents

William C. Menninger	1946-51
Sol W. Ginsburg	1955-57

PUBLICATIONS BOARD

Chairman

Ronald M. Wintrob, M.D.
McCook Hospital
2 Holcomb Street
Hartford, Conn. 06112

Margaret M. Lawrence
Carl P. Malmquist
Alfred H. Stanton
Herbert Weiner

Consultant
Melvin Sabshin

ex Officio
Judd Marmor
Gene L. Usdin
Jack A. Wolford

COMMITTEE ACKNOWLEDGMENTS

The Committee on Therapeutic Care is indebted to the following persons who participated in the formulation of this report: to Ian L. W. Clancey, at that time a member of the Committee; to Robert L. Jimenez and Andrea Delgado, Ginsburg Fellows assigned to the Committee, 1971-72 and 1973-74, respectively, who also assisted in the Committee's work; and to Helen F. Hough of the Editorial Staff of the Mental Health Materials Center for her invaluable assistance in organizing and editing the report. To these and to others, in the field, without whose vital cooperation this report could not have been completed, the Committee is grateful.

INTRODUCTION

With the emergence of the community mental health movement and the emphasis on community-based treatment, a whole new system for the delivery of human services is developing in this country. Much of the care in this system will be provided by community workers (outreach workers, neighborhood workers, indigenous workers) who perhaps number more than 100,000, and represent the largest influx of manpower into the mental health field in any single decade.

Originally conceived as a solution to the manpower problem, later supported as a method of employing the poor, and at times advocated as an instrument of social and institutional change, community workers have begun to demonstrate their value by communicating and working with populations and problems relatively inaccessible to traditional mental health personnel. In the course of their activities they have extended the concept of mental health to encompass the totality of human services. They respond to unmet human needs and human deprivations in all the intersecting systems in which community life is enmeshed—health, education, welfare, housing, jobs, and law enforcement. They also address themselves to institutional change as exemplified by problems created by poverty, racism, elitism, and professionalism.

Despite the crucial involvement of community workers in providing services, little has been documented of the range and scope of their activities, the extent of their patient/client involvement, or the nature of their interventions. Because of the intrinsic importance of the subject, the Committee on Therapeutic Care undertook a study and description of the different kinds of neighborhood workers and the varieties of their training; a conceptualization of their views of human behavior and their methods of intervention; and an analysis of the range and scope of their activities and of the issues they raise.

Data for the study were obtained by visits to 13 carefully selected neighborhood health centers (see Appendix Table 1), where on-site discussions were held with staff personnel and their records examined. There were also discussions with the workers, who welcomed our accompanying them on home visits. Committee members later reviewed these activities with them in order to understand the reasons for their helping behavior. Members also read extensively in the literature, as well as drawing upon direct experiences from their own clinical settings.

The methods used and the data obtained impose certain limitations on the inferences to be drawn and the conclusions reached in this report (see Appendix Table 2). As a result, the Committee cannot adequately describe the dynamics of these workers' interactions with individuals, families and groups over time. The data are simply not comparable in richness and depth to those obtained from the observations of residents in similar situations. The workers' responses to the poignant predicaments of their clients is direct, action-oriented, and focused on the manifest content of reality-induced stresses. Hence the attempt to conceptualize their experience in terms of "A Sense of Human Need: The Worker's Model" (Section 1). This model is of a different order of conceptualization from our customary bio-psycho-social, or psychobiological, or developmental psychodynamic models. In consequence, these models are not comparable. The workers' model and the professional models are of different orders of abstraction.

Nor did the Committee undertake an analysis of all the tasks with which mental health personnel are confronted, the organization and structuring of work tasks, and the knowledge and skills necessary for their performance. Work and task analysis would permit a more accurate assessment of the worker's virtues and limitations (as well as the professional's) and of what workers have to contribute to professionals in understanding and skills. Functions and roles could then be defined in terms of tasks, and hence would be more amenable to measurement, determination of cost effectiveness, certification, and evaluation.

1

A SENSE OF HUMAN NEED: THE WORKER'S MODEL

The community worker tends to view the basic cause of his patient's* difficulty as deriving, not from inner stress, but from external deprivation as rooted in the inequities of the social and economic order in our country. A recognition of this viewpoint of the etiology of his patient's distress is essential to understanding the interactions the worker undertakes.

A similar viewpoint has recently been expressed by a past president of the American Psychiatric Association.† Dr. Busse expressed his view of the inseparable relationship between human health and socioeconomic well-being as follows:

> Since World War II, there has been a gradual change in social values. A number of what have been considered privileges and sometimes luxuries are now recognized as basic human needs. . . . I do not believe that the health problem is separable from the total social-economic situation for some minorities. The discrepancy between the majority and certain subgroups in life span, as well as the extent of disability and illnesses, is not related primarily to the absence of a comprehensive health care system. It is even more determined by adverse social-economic conditions that have often resulted directly, as well as indirectly, in irreversible damage to the health of the individual.

In the Committee's contacts with community workers, members found that workers conceptualized their patients'

* The word *client* is used by workers with equal frequency.

† Ewald W. Busse, M.D., speaking at the 23rd Annual Institute of Hospital and Community Psychiatry held in Seattle, Washington, 1971.

problems as stemming from the frustration of basic human (psychologic, social and physiologic) needs. Those factors which seemed to interfere with the gratification of these human needs were perceived by the workers as primarily social and economic in origin. In effect, the workers perceived their clients and their communities as victimized by cultural and situational forces somewhat beyond their immediate control.

As the workers viewed their clients' distress from their unique vantage point (one perhaps differing from that of many health professionals), they saw basic human needs frustrated by overwhelming external forces. They therefore tended to conceptualize these events in terms reflecting a heightened sense of the urgency and reality-oriented nature of their clients' needs. The Committee has tried through case examples provided by community workers to use this concept of need as an approach to understanding the interaction between those who signal distress and those who respond to it.

The nature of some of these interchanges is illustrated through the use of brief clinical vignettes. Some of these clinical examples clearly reveal that the patient's plea for help was made while he was in a situation of acute crisis, often expressed as a distinctly personal (individual) need or dilemma, but often an expression of family (group) turmoil and disorganization. Other examples indicate that the complaints or pleas of the patients were an expression of long-standing unresolved conflict and deprivation having complex emotional and socioeconomic determinants.

The following outline and examples were derived from interviews held by Committee members with community workers in a variety of community settings. The word *need* is related to the usual "chief complaint," as expressed by the individual patient. *Need* suggests, however, a broader interpersonal and social context than any specific complaint. This concept seemed useful in summarizing, via the case examples, *the situations of deprivation as seen through the eyes of the community worker.* As can be verified from the case examples, these situations do not always lend themselves neatly or exclusively to any particular grouping in outline form. Nevertheless, to the extent that the group headings, within the Committee's outline of needs-deprivations provide a basic framework for description and reference, they will have accomplished their purpose:

OUTLINE: Needs Rooted in Deprivations That Are Followed by Loss of Security

- I. Need for Milieu Reliability
  - A. Dependability of relationships
  - B. Cultural sustenance
- II. Need for Boundary Definition and Permeability
  - A. Reality orientation
  - B. Problem-solving assistance
- III. Need for Personal Fulfillment
  - A. Freedom of expression and choice
  - B. Role continuity and evolution
- IV. Need for Performance Rewards
  - A. Opportunity for achievement
  - B. Group attention and affirmation

CASE EXAMPLES: Origin and Use

The numbered case examples represent a highly condensed, and therefore perhaps oversimplified, statement of the most immediately presenting problem as expressed by the patient and as formulated by the workers. The more detailed exposition and definition of the various "needs" are in turn derived from the reports and from the clinical data provided by the workers, who were interviewed by members of the Committee. These case examples are grouped according to the presenting or predominant need at the time of initial patient contact with the community worker.

OUTLINE NEED I (for Milieu Reliability)

Within the need for milieu reliability (Need I in the outline preceding), dependability of relationships (A) ranks as an uppermost factor. Dependability of relationships suggests a need for the feeling of constancy, belonging, and continuity in living with others.

A—Dependability of relationships

Case example #1. A 14-year-old girl phoned a "Drop in" center. She was frightened and hesitant, at first talking in generalities. Finally she mentioned her use of "speed." Her parents had not given her their support in seeking help, nor did they acknowledge the existence of a problem. They disapproved of the Center because of the "Hippie style" dress of clinic personnel, its clients, and its association with "addicts." The girl was thinking of suicide. (See also Section 5, Case example #1.)

Case example #2. Both parents in a family with 7 children were alcoholics. The mother had attempted suicide and had left home, with her children, to live with another man. The father wanted his children back but was unable to claim them despite the fact that the mother neglected them. When the police threatened the mother with taking her children away from her, she threatened in retaliation to kill the worker!

Case example #3. A 40-year-old man known to a worker for several years said he needed a job. The worker was aware that his client's wife had left him. Since that time he appeared not to care about anything. He looked sad and depressed, lacked confidence, and seemed without a life purpose or any feeling of personal worth.

These cases emphasize the need for environmental constancy, for durable sharing with significant persons—parents, spouse, children, friends, teachers, clergyman, supervisor. They imply the need to feel part of a group (family, peer, work), to feel acknowledged and cared for by others, the need for models to offer guidance, protection, support, interest, care and stimulation. Such needs convey the importance of basic family and other social values in a rapidly changing world.

B—Cultural sustenance

This implies the need for quite specific kinds of support in the areas of

1) Health.
2) Training, that is, a usable vocational skill that will contribute to the maintenance of the family, home, and community.
3) A stable source of income for the purchase of food, clothing, shelter.
4) A variety of coping skills to make possible communication, learning, teaching, sharing and nurturing.
5) Friendly contacts for solace and companionship.
6) Assistance and advice on matters monetary, vocational and legal.
7) A system of values, ethics and laws gained from models for utilization in developing parental guidance, authority, and family integrity.

Case example #4. A community worker knocked on a neighborhood door and found a family living on welfare payments. Father and son both needed jobs. The father was sick "with back trouble."

Case example #5. The occupants of one dwelling said they were not in need of help, but as they talked, the worker learned that the husband and wife were both alcoholics (see also Section 5, Case example #5). The husband had no job and the wife was crippled. They had no money for food or rent.

Case example #6. A 55-year-old single white woman with cerebral palsy who lived alone was found by a black worker. The woman walked with difficulty and spoke so poorly that she could hardly be understood. Her home was cluttered, dirty, and inadequately furnished. Minimally she seemed to need money and a doctor, but hadn't been able to mobilize herself to obtain help.

These cases illustrate the frequency of multiple problems, especially the relationship of health problems to other needs for cultural sustenance.

OUTLINE NEED II (for Boundary Definition and Permeability)

A—Reality orientation

Orientation to reality involves clarification and interpretation of key parameters of one's life as these relate to all components of the family and the community. This includes —

1) Confirmation of the reality of time, place, and person.
2) An understanding of the meaning and nature of one's tasks in the family, in the home, and at work; and a reasonable assignment and performance of tasks.
3) The means for cooperative interaction and constructive resolution of conflicts about roles and tasks.
4) Recognition and acknowledgment of the needs, strengths and weaknesses in oneself and others.
5) The assurance of dependability in others.
6) The capacity for identification, imitation, and separation.
7) Some assessment of human and material resources in the environment that are relevant to one's needs and available for their satisfaction.

Worker's report a. "I have met any number of mothers who appear to require more attention, guidance and just plain old-fashioned mothering than the children they are attempting to rear. For whatever reason, they cannot seem to get into common everyday routines like feeding the children or getting them off to school every day at the right time. They seem to have no real conception of time and often do not allow the time for the shopping that must be done or the meals that ought to be planned. They have never set up any clear-cut rules for the children—when to go to bed, when to eat, where to play, etc. One woman I know was concerned about recreation for her 8-year-old son, but she was so confused about how to handle it that she actually took him out dancing until two o'clock in the morning! She told me she felt obligated to 'do things' with her children."

Worker's report b. "I decided it would help the neighborhood if I started a girl's group for fifth graders through junior high. The contacts were made by the mothers, who seemed to resent me at first. Then they openly admitted they were having difficulties with the children in various areas—mostly acting out sexually, with some shoplifting, smoking and that sort of thing. But they didn't know what to do about their situation. These mothers, I felt, were genuinely interested in their daughters, but sadly enough they seemed to be perpetuating the difficulties that were giving the most trouble. Some of them knew what their problems were, and some of them even knew what was needed, but all of them seemed to feel powerless to initiate the kind of communication with their daughters that would close the gap between them."

B—Problem-solving assistance

This calls for ready access to people who can provide support, and help in solving problems of group living. The underlying need suggests that assistance is necessary in evaluating and responding to tension-inducing situations so that tensions (inner and outer) may be resolved. Personnel whose assistance would be valuable are those who (1) can provide counsel within or for the family; (2) can define and clarify the socioeconimic interface between the family and the community; or (3) have a good working knowledge of the human and social resources in the community.

Case example #7. A 21-year-old man came to a community center and asked for help with drug addiction. The worker who talked with him learned that he was a compulsive gambler who had been involved with criminals. The patient was extremely anxious and seemed on the verge of psychosis. His father was an alcoholic. His oldest brother had killed himself several years before by pouring kerosene over himself and igniting it.

Worker's report c. "The immediate need of my clients in more than a few cases is just a matter of transportation. They need to go see a doctor, or they need to get home from some place but don't have the carfare to get back. Their children need to be taken to school but where they have their own car, they don't have the gasoline, or the snow tires, or the car just won't start."

Case example #8. The worker was asked to see a 16-year-old girl, a high school senior, in a crisis clinic. The girl had swallowed a number of pills in a suicidal gesture and felt she had problems she needed help in understanding. Several years previously she had been abandoned by her mother, an alcoholic, and had since been living with an older sister of 23, who had recently married. Her father had left the family when the patient was 3 years old and had not been heard from since. (See also Section 2, Case example #8.)

The girl felt she was a loner. Her behavior and performance at school had only intensified her sense of isolation and worthlessness. The pill-swallowing episode served to draw attention to her predicament. The worker intervened to assist her in understanding that the pill-swallowing episode served as a method of drawing attention to her predicament.

OUTLINE NEED III (for Personal Fulfillment)

A—Freedom of expression and choice

Gratification of this need allows the expression and exchange of affection, love, regard, and respect through both agreement and disagreement. It flourishes in the absence of harassment by people, poverty, danger, illness, or fear. It suggests the universal human need to communicate what one feels, to be understood and acknowledged, and to receive a meaningful response. It asserts the individual freedom to imagine, choose, act, approach or retreat, believe or disbelieve, assume or relinquish responsibility, reveal or conceal.

Case example #9. A black worker was making case-finding calls in her neighborhood. One white woman in her late twenties, Mrs. N, who had 8 children, all with her, lived in 3 cold rooms which had no adequate source of heat. A table, a bed, a chair and an old couch comprised the only furniture. The children slept on the floor. The husband was living in another city and had last sent home $50 about 3 months before. Mrs. N was not receiving welfare payments, had little food and no money. Her youngest children, who were 3-month-old twins, had the appearance of newborns. The only food available for them was a box of oatmeal. The woman herself was ill, as were 2 of her children. She had been afraid to apply for welfare because she knew this would entail her swearing out a warrant against her husband and she feared he might return and harm her. She felt trapped.

Mrs. N was assisted in seeing that her interpretation of her situation had been unnecessarily rigid and that genuine alternatives were available to her (see also Section 2, Case example #9).

Case example #10. A 36-year-old woman sought help from a worker in coping with her husband's "lack of understanding." She was the mother of 9 children and had had 4 postpartum depressions. In 12 years of marriage her husband had had 8 geographical job transfers. The last child had been born 10 months before the interview. Shortly after the birth, her husband announced another transfer. She resented his "cruel and cutting remarks" about her inability to cope and expressed the feeling that he had "taken advantage" of her.

At the very least in this case, there was the need for both husband and wife to understand the intensity of stress that they were both experiencing. This is typical of the cases the community worker encounters.

B—Role continuity and evolution

This need to experience a sense of satisfaction, usefulness, and regard accrues over a period of time from successful assumption of roles in the family and the community. Satisfaction is less dependent on technical proficiency than it is on interpersonal adequacy in establishing and maintaining certain key roles—friendship, marital, parental, and so on. Gratification is rather dependent on such complex processes as imitation, and implies the availability of suitable models who provide the support and guidance needed for optimum personality development and maturation.

Case example #11. A 17-year-old Puerto Rican youth, newly arrived on the continent, entered a community mental health center seeking employment. The worker learned that he spoke no English, had no friends, and no knowledge of work opportunities in the area.

Case example #12. A 35-year-old black college graduate was brought to a day center by his parents, who were concerned about his withdrawal. The man himself had no clear complaint. He did not "want to be at home" and did "want a job." The patient conveyed feelings of suppressed hostility and seemed to have no channel for the expression of such feelings, except drinking to excess in an effort to wall them off (see Section 2, Case example #12).

These two cases, though different, both illustrate the need for assistance in establishing a role within the community and the need for a sense of satisfaction and usefulness.

OUTLINE NEED IV (for Performance Rewards)

A—Opportunity for achievement

This implies the day-to-day exercise of a skill for which one has been trained or educated to the point of technical competency. It implies also a wish or need to aspire to excellence of performance. The sense of achievement is related to the successful completion of a task, which in turn insures the reciprocal response by a feeling of self-confidence, accomplishment and personal worth. Thus the satisfaction of this need engenders feelings of (1) continuing hope, meaning, zest, adequacy, well-being and creativity in life; (2) preparedness in oneself for carrying out a useful role in the family and community; and (3) a just relationship between having contributed and having been rewarded by life.

Case example #13. A 17-year-old Puerto Rican youth inflicted cigarette burns on his 1-year-old nephew. The mother of the burned baby sought treatment for his burns from a nearby community health clinic. The clinic worker (a 23-year-old divorced Puerto Rican mother of 2 children) arranged to interview the youth, who had been living with his brother and sister-in-law in a small apartment ever since his unannounced arrival in this country 3 months previously.

The worker discovered that the youth was frustrated, lonely and quite depressed at his inability to obtain employment (see also Section 5, Case example #13). His history revealed recent severe head trauma (skull fracture) and treatment with anticonvulsant medication. This boy felt misunderstood and unwanted, and he had reacted with violence to what he perceived as an inhospitable, intolerable environment. He resented the attention being paid his nephew whom he burned "in retaliation."

B—Group attention and affirmation

This implies that one's feeling of self-regard is enhanced in a group (family, work, peer) whose members have reason to exchange evidences of regard for one another. Such a group enjoys free expressions of interest, concern, and care. In effect, the group setting promotes the experience of closeness, reasonable competition, kindliness, cooperation, compromise, and the enjoyment of play, mobility, and friendship.

Case example #14. An active, likable man 72 years of age and one of the worker's lifelong personal friends asked her for help in getting a job. His wife had died. He felt lonely and craved companionship.

Contact with the worker in this instance assuaged this man's feelings of isolation and paved the way for group contacts of a supporting nature.

Case example #15. A worker was asked to help with the problems of a family of 4—father, mother, and 2 daughters aged 12 and 4 years. The mother said, "I'm having trouble with my 12-year-old—can't control her. She's pregnant and she won't listen to us."

The father had no job, few friends, and he had abdicated responsibility. The mother did not regard herself as feminine or appealing. She felt lonely and unable to make the home attractive or even livable. The 4-year-old seemed not to be getting sufficient guidance from anyone. All seemed to share the feeling of isolation.

Many interventions and resources were required and many resources mobilized to alter this situation (see Section 2, Case example #15, for resources and interventions utilized to resolve these problems).

Reality orientation of the worker

The community worker's activity can best be understood, in the opinion of this committee, when one appreciates the particular viewpoint of the worker toward his client's suffering. The worker tends on the whole to see his patient's need for help as the consequence of powerful and even overwhelming external forces which act to frustrate a gamut of basic human needs. These needs are then perceived by the worker as urgently requiring an immediate, reality-oriented resolution. This is not to deny that some community workers, especially those with formal training, have and do operate within a more traditional, internally focused, psychodynamic view of their patients' difficulties.

2

PATTERNS AND PRINCIPLES OF THE WORKER'S INTERVENTIONS

In the reassessment of the health needs in our country, attention has been focused on the reorganization of the health care system to improve delivery of service and on the selection and training of new classes of health workers. Little or no attention has been given to the kinds of services actually being delivered to the recipient. It was the intent of the Committee on Therapeutic Care to focus on the transaction between the community purveyor and the neighborhood consumer of the health services. Interest was appropriately focused on this transaction inasmuch as our clinical orientation had previously led us to explore a similar transaction in the hospital setting between the nursing staff and the patient.

In our survey of the hospital transaction we were able to delineate certain principles of therapeutic interaction which were summarized in GAP Report No. 77, TOWARD THERAPEUTIC CARE.[1] It appeared desirable to explore the possibility that similar or related principles were operating in the community health setting. If they were, it would be of value to delineate these principles and illustrate them with meaningful case examples.

The field survey providing the data discussed in this report strengthened our conviction that the transactions taking place at the interface between the community worker and the patient/client are sufficiently important and even crucial to the well-being of the latter to warrant further investigation. The physical setting is certainly different (the transaction was in the home rather than the hospital), but the needs expressed by the patient/client and the help offered by the worker seemed quite comparable to what may be seen in the hospital. To verify the belief that the nature of these findings by and large reflected what was taking place in the neighborhood centers across the country, each member of the Committee visited centers in his home community (Appendix Table 1). There he interviewed agency leaders and workers, compiled information about the neighborhood service, and, through selected case vignettes, attempted to capture the quality of the transaction between worker and client. (The format utilized for gathering these data is reproduced in Appendix Table 2 of this report.)

It is fair to say that the problems cited by the workers in the health agencies surveyed bear out the current view of the social and health problems that have been vigorously discussed (if perhaps less vigorously pursued) by government agencies in the past few years. In brief, the community workers were of the opinion that housing, education, employment, food, health (prevention and treatment), and drug and alcohol addiction were all major problems. They felt that their patient-clients were significantly uninformed about the range and kinds of services available and that this was at least in part due to the cultural deprivation of these patient-clients.

The workers also felt that in far too many cases the agencies set up expressly to assist their patient-clients utilized procedures inappropriately or excessively to limit the services actually given. Likewise they felt that agencies were so poorly coordinated that considerably less than optimal service was provided. Surprisingly, race as a problem was not accorded the same urgency in discussion as problems of housing, education, employment, food, or health.

The workers are in rather clear agreement about what is helpful in assisting their patient-clients to solve their problems. *In general, those procedures which assist their patient-clients in becoming independent (autonomous) members of the community were considered the most helpful.* These procedures were regarded as tangible rather than intangible. For example, if a man is unemployed, get him a job or get him training that will have a job as its payoff; if an individual or a family has no place to live, get them a place to live and the economic wherewithal to remain there; if a mother has to get to a doctor, make transportation and baby-sitting services available.

Certainly there were other areas of assistance which community workers felt were useful. For example, they felt that providing information was helpful—that is, information to children and parents about such issues as homemaking, nutrition, how to negotiate with the community for specific services needed. They were further of the opinion that the increase in their patient-clients' self-awareness resulting from the worker's role as sounding board in a friendship relation fostered the move toward autonomy, which they considered the crucial objective. Encouraging their patient-clients to engage in social activities and constructive projects in the community also in their view supported the patient-clients' commitment to independence. These activities seemed to the workers to foster a meaningful positive relationship with others which made their patient-clients more effective and hopeful.

The workers made an effort to define specifically what they saw as their patient-clients' major problems (needs) and to characterize their own approach to the resolution of these problems (meeting the needs). Problems were generally perceived as real and as external. The worker conceptualized his role in meeting these problems as equally realistic, although he often conceptualized to committee members the hoped-for result in more abstract terms (e.g., to achieve autonomy).

It should be noted that a need-oriented action did not characterize the working style of the full range of community workers. The less trained tended to use a need-fulfilling, relatively less dynamic model in conceptualizing their work. The worker having more traditional training used a more dynamic conceptualization and was relatively less action-oriented in his approach to his work.

In reviewing the case vignettes provided by the workers, the

Committee sought concepts which would capture the nature of the worker's interventions and describe in concrete terms his link to the immediate and real world in which he functions. It seemed to the Committee members that most of the interventions of the worker vis à vis his patient/client could be subsumed under one or more of the following activity categories:*

1) Solving problems of *deprivation* by providing food, clothing, or shelter.
2) Relaxing *family tensions* by getting a family member treatment for an illness, rearranging family sleeping arrangements and the like.
3) Providing *education* (e.g., in homemaking skills, or helping a client return to school).
4) Arranging for *expert counsel* (physician, lawyer).
5) Assisting in *changing the environment*—for example, by helping the patient move to suitable quarters.
6) Supporting a sense of *social leverage, effectiveness or linkage* (such as helping a needy client get on welfare).
7) Removing *noxious stimuli* (e.g., lead paint from a child's home).
8) Encouraging *internal resolution* of personal problems (e.g., worker as a model—"be like me").

All these activities were perceived by the worker as fostering the independence of his patient/client.

TYPICAL INTERVENTIONS

Case example #16 (Mrs. B) interventions

The following is a detailed and verbatim account of a response by an outreach worker who functions as part of a demonstration health project in a city department of health. The project objective was to upgrade the health of children in an economically depressed area. The interaction between this worker and

* The intervention techniques are potentially useful in meeting any or all of the need categories previously described.

her client characterizes many of the interventions previously mentioned: solving problems of deprivation, education, arranging expert counsel, supporting a sense of effectiveness, and fostering internal resolution of personal conflicts.

Worker's report d. Mrs. B was referred to me by the nurse. She had "worked up" this family and had brought the kids in for screening and physicals. For some reason or other she felt she couldn't get close to this woman, so she asked me if I would make some home visits with her. After going with her a couple of times, I built up a relationship with this woman and was able to get close to Mrs. B, who had 5 children.

Mrs. B lived with her mother, sisters and brothers in a 3-bedroom home that would have been adequate probably for a family of 6, but 13 people were living in the house at the time I started visiting. Mrs. B had not been able to get any welfare. She was told that because she lived in the house with her parents, they were responsible for her.

Mrs. B was 36 years old. Her children had many medical needs and she felt there was something wrong with herself as well. She complained of having "spells" where she would black out and couldn't breathe. She knew she had had rheumatic fever as a child but felt there was no money she could honestly spend on a doctor for herself.

Mrs. B defined her total needs as medical services for the children and herself, and financial help. She reported feeling "very bad having to depend on my family for everything the children get," yet she knew of no other way their needs might be taken care of. I saw Mrs. B's needs as not only medical care for herself and the children but also adequate housing away from her family, plus the money to take care of her own personal needs.

We started by making an appointment with the welfare office together. Upon getting there we were told that no money could be allotted Mrs. B until she moved out of her parents' home. We tried every means we could think of to find a house. We even had some money donated to us to pay the first month's rent, but Mrs. B was reluctant to leave home. I think possibly most of her reluctance was due to her fear that she couldn't quite manage the job of taking care of the children with her own health in such a poor state.

Mrs. B herself was seen by Dr. Z at the hospital because we were concerned and felt we couldn't wait until the welfare people decided to help her. Dr. Z volunteered to see her and after doing so decided that she did have a cardiac condition calling for medical attention. He promptly admitted her to the hospital, ran a number of tests, and then called the welfare department to report his opinion that it was very important for her to be given a medical card. As a result of his intervention, Mrs. B was given a medical card and money to help her meet expenses of the children.

Of course, with Mrs. B's kids living in our area, we could take care of their medical needs. Upon examination they were found to have anemia, bad teeth, and many psychological problems probably brought on by the overcrowded conditions in their grandparents' home and by Mrs. B's low self-esteem, plus many other problems within the family. The kids, ages 10 and 8, had dropped off in their school work. We felt it was probably because there were so many women in this home bossing them around. The boys couldn't really grow up without some male figure to relate to. After I had worked with Mrs. B for a while, she herself mentioned that she realized this was a problem and at that point she started trying to get men involved with the kids—like her brother and her uncle. In the past two years these boys have really come out of it.

We still haven't been able to get Mrs. B to move out of her parents' home. However, sisters and brothers have moved out since, so that the house is less crowded than it used to be. Also, Mrs. B did go back to school through Vocational Rehabilitation and got some training as a secretary. She was unable to find employment even after going to school because she felt they didn't teach her enough and the school hadn't taught her what most employers expect their secretaries to know. She is employed now part time as a sales clerk.

Things are much better in this home now. The children are happier and their medical needs are being met. No one has to go and visit now. Mrs. B is able to stand alone, and whenever she needs help she knows where to call and just what it is that she needs.

I started working with Mrs. B about 3 years ago and there were many times when her spirits were low. In fact, there were times when she would call me in the middle of the night. She was being pressured by her family to file charges against her husband, to whom she was still very much tied. Welfare was also asking her to file papers against him. This woman was feeling such mixed emotions that she didn't know what to do. At one point in our visiting, she mentioned that she had even thought about suicide. I tried talking with her and found it more than I could handle. Upon talking with my supervisor, we did get her an appointment at the State Hospital Outpatient Department. I went with her on this first visit and I think they set her up for two more appointments. After completing her appointments Mrs. B was told that she had every right to feel very low and they didn't consider her a candidate for the State Hospital. She has called me many times since to say that she was thinking of suicide but in the last year she has not called at all.

I do feel that Mrs. B is on the upturn and is now able to take care of her children. I am going with her now to get her teeth pulled. She is going to take sodium pentathol and would like to have somebody with her.

Comments. This client's problem was first identified by a nurse in the project. She in turn asked the help of the community worker because of her inability to establish rapport with the client. The nurse and the worker then made joint home visits to permit the latter to develop a relationship with the client. The problems the worker identified were (1) inadequate housing, (2) the need for public financial support, and (3) the need of the client and her children for medical attention. The worker then proceeded with the following program: (a) to correct existing deprivations, (b) to educate Mrs. B in ways both formal (to attend school for job training) and informal (personal discussion), (c) to solicit effective professional counsel from a physician and a psychiatrist for her client, and (d) to utilize social leverage (by putting pressure on the welfare department) to improve the social effectiveness of the client. Only the worker's attempt to change the environmental locale of the family by making it possible for them to move was unsuccessful.

Case example #9 (Mrs. N) interventions

Mrs. N and her children were first seen by a community worker employed in a multiservice neighborhood agency funded by the Model Cities Program (see Case example #9 in

Section 1 preceding). The agency services the major poverty area of the city in which it is located. The following report of the worker's activities describes the effect of correcting serious family deprivation, providing education, and reversing the overriding sense of hopelessness that characterizes so many families in need. The continued interest of the worker contributed significantly to a positive result.

A warrant was required by the welfare department before Mrs. N could be certified for support payments, but the worker got her own supervisor to come with her that day. Together they were able to get emergency clothing and food for Mrs. N and her family. They used agency transportation to take Mrs. N's 2 sick children to the hospital (one child, who had pneumonia, was hospitalized between 4 and 6 weeks, the other, who had hepatitis, for 2 months).

The worker and her supervisor moved a bed into Mrs. N's lodgings that day and the following day got two more beds, and bedsheets. Their sources of supply were the agency and some residents in the neighborhood. She and her supervisor put up $7 between them to buy Mrs. N a stove. The outreach worker then called a local charity center, which sent someone over with beans, canned goods, oatmeal and peaches, and also clothes and shoes.

In the weeks that followed, the worker persuaded Mrs. N to sign the necessary warrant against her husband. Welfare had initially instructed her to go to New York to sign the form. Meanwhile the worker and her supervisor had obtained a food and rent voucher from the welfare department for her. The vouchers have continued.

In 2 months, Mrs. N got her first check from Welfare, which she showed to the outreach worker, thinking she had to pay the agency back for what they had done. Now she has a new stove, new living room furniture, a washing machine, and bunkbeds for the children. She was helped by the agency to get her high school diploma. Currently she has put her small children in the day care center while she attends school to become a practical nurse.

Mrs. N moved with her children to another area to avoid her husband, who had returned from New York. She is doing very well. The agency contact had lasted 14 months. The worker felt that she was still hung up by her fear of her husband.

Comments. The client was identified as in need of help by the worker, who had met her during a routine round of knocking on doors to get acquainted and inform the neighbors of the services of her agency. She saw at once the need of Mrs. N and her 8 children for food, furniture, medical attention, and financial assistance. Her major interventions were the mobilization of personal and social resources to correct deprivations and to obtain expert counsel in the form of medical services for the children. Using her relationship with her client, the worker was able to assist in providing Mrs. N an educational opportunity which in turn permitted her to move her home and thereby avoid disturbing contact with her estranged husband.

Case example #17 interventions

An indigenous community worker was involved by a physician on the medical staff of her agency in an attempt to alter the noxious environment of a patient/client and her 3 fatherless children. The worker focused her efforts on helping the mother make her apartment safe for her children. When this failed, the worker and mother together sought out ways to find a new and safer place for the family to live.

Worker's report e. The oldest child in the family, a girl of 5, was found on routine examination to be suffering from lead poisoning. The source of the lead was the paint on the walls of the apartment in which they were living.

A plan of action was developed by the community worker, the physician, and the mother to eliminate this dangerous poison from the child's environment.

1) The worker called the City Building Inspection Unit, which made an inspection of the apartment and notified the landlord that he was in violation of the building code. The landlord's response was to paper the walls of the apartment. Unfortunately, the child continued to eat the lead paint, scraping the paper off the walls to get at it. As the source of the lead paint remained, the worker, through a nurse she knew, made a contact with Legal Aid, whose representative checked the condition of the apartment. As he was of the opinion that a problem did exist, the Society filed suit against the building owner which is still pending.

2) Because of their concern about the continued exposure of the child to the lead, the worker, the nurse, and the child's mother are currently considering a move to new quarters. Contacts have been made with the Housing Authority and again with Legal Aid to work on the possibility that this family might obtain public housing.

3) During this period the child has been under treatment for lead poisoning and on two occasions has required hospitalization. Currently her condition is reported as greatly improved. A new apartment, free of lead paint, is in the offing for this family.

Comments. The child was identified as in need of help at the time of a routine physical examination. Her problem clearly called for removal of a noxious chemical agent (lead) from her environment. The community worker was able to mobilize the social forces—City Building Inspection Unit, Legal Aid, and Housing Authority—to effect a practical improvement in the child's physical environment.

Case example #15 interventions

(see also Section 1, Case example #15)

The community worker for a neighborhood agency effectively mobilized the energies of a family toward greater independence. Her use of herself as a role model, although largely effective, seems to have disadvantaged one member of the family, the mother. This is an occasional risk secondary to the explicit nature of the interventions of the community worker. The initial contact had been made through a welfare worker, who requested help with a family of 4—mother, father and 2 daughters 12 and 4 years old. The parents' concern was their 12-year-old daughter, whom they couldn't control ("She's pregnant and she won't listen to us").

The worker felt that a number of problems existed in the family. The father was not taking an active role in family life and was abdicating responsibility. He was out of a job. The mother was not viewing herself as a woman ("not keeping herself appealing") and was not aware of the many things she could do to make the home a more livable place. The 12-year-old, who was bright and active, was not getting precise role models from mother or father.

The worker directed her interventions toward several areas. She instructed the mother in home management techniques; offered her "tips" on how to make herself more attractive. She assisted the father in finding a job and became involved with the 12-year-old daughter.

Response was varied: The father responded to the assertiveness and resourcefulness of the worker by viewing her interventions as demonstrating qualities his wife didn't have. The mother felt threatened by the worker. The daughter identified the worker as the mother she needed and wanted. The worker felt she was becoming "too involved" with the family and sought, by replacing herself with another worker who would function differently with the family, to minimize the tension engendered. Nevertheless she felt she had accomplished several desirable objectives:

1) Laid the basic groundwork for future intervention.
2) Put in some of the "dirty work" that had to be done in order to continue working with this family.
3) Helped with home management by minimizing discussion of personal problems; realistically defined her

purpose and function by actually telling clients, "This is not my role," or "I cannot discuss this, but we can discuss that," etc.

4) Coordinated agencies in assisting the family, and in general changed the emphasis of the various agency functions from a custodial one in which the family's behavior was viewed as pathological to one in which the family was viewed as a family that could function with help.
5) Brought in a male worker to help the father.

Comments. This family was referred by a welfare worker because the mother had expressed concern over "controlling" her pregnant 12-year-old daughter. The community worker saw other needs: (a) for the father to be more active and responsible, (b) for the mother to be more appealing as a woman and more effective as a homemaker, (c) for the daughter to see in mother and father more explicit, positive people. Accordingly the worker tried to educate the mother in homemaking and personal grooming while helping the father get a job. Although she tried to avoid overinvolvement, she did recognize that this was occurring and withdrew in favor of a male worker. The unfortunate aspect of the worker's transactions with the family was that they increased family tensions by suggesting to both father and daughter comparisons between her and the mother wherein they openly preferred the worker over the mother. An alternative that would have mobilized the entire family, including the mother, would of course have been more desirable.

Case example #8 (Miss S) interventions

(see also Section 1, Case example #8)

The following describes the activities of a worker who has received training. The interaction is of a different order from that of the indigenous untrained neighborhood worker. We see a mental health technician working in a crisis clinic. The problem is conceptualized as psychological and subjective. The intervention used is "talking" with the patient/client in order to raise the level of her self-awareness.

The initial contact with this adolescent patient was made in the Crisis Clinic after she had swallowed a number of pills in a suicidal gesture. Miss S was quite cooperative. She arrived at the Clinic with her brother-in-law and in the interview saw herself as needing help in understanding and dealing with her problems and her feelings. The interviewer was in agreement with the client on the basis of the history that she and her brother-in-law gave. Miss S did in fact have a number of problems which needed to be resolved. One of the most urgent needs of this patient was that of forming a relationship with another person and gaining some understanding of the demands placed by such a relationship on herself as well as on the other party.

At 16, Miss S was a senior in high school. She was living with her 23-year-old sister and brother-in-law since abandonment at 13 by her mother. The mother is a chronic alcoholic and had not been very helpful in dealing with any type of problem. The father had abandoned the family when Miss S was 3 years old, and has not been heard from since. The patient is the youngest of 4 children. She seemed to find it very difficult to relate to the worker and described herself in a quite negative way as being a loner very self-conscious around other people. There have been school problems over the past 2 years, because she defies any authority and has been verbally abusive both at home and at school.

Miss S was seen over a period of 5 months in individual treatment on a weekly basis. At first, the main focus was on forming a relationship with the therapist. This proved most difficult for the patient and took a great deal of time. The second objective was to enable her to perceive that she created most of her difficulties and that something specific could be done about this.

Interventions were achieved with the cooperation of Miss S

as well as through the school and her family. There was a good deal of contact with all of them. Miss S was in need of continuing therapy and consequently was referred to the outpatient service of a local hospital, where she is currently being seen on a weekly basis. The intervention that was made has helped her in a number of ways. Having completed high school, she is now holding down a full-time job. She has gotten in touch with the worker in an effort to continue a relationship that was very difficult to form and has proved equally difficult to terminate.

Comment. In the case of Miss S, she was brought to a crisis clinic by her brother-in-law after a suicidal gesture. The initial focus was on forming a relationship with the worker. The second area for exploration was the patient's contribution to her problems. Interventions were made in the home and at school. The patient improved and was referred for more extended psychological treatment. It is clear that the interaction of the more highly trained worker in this case is not that of the indigenous worker. The point is not that the interaction is better or worse but rather that it is different. The worker in this case was clearly using a psychotherapeutic procedure to carry out her task.

Case example #12 interventions
(see also Section 1, Case example #12)

The worker in this case was an art therapist working in a day treatment center. She conceptualized her function along the traditional lines of a hospital-based activities therapist. She worked effectively and smoothly, but not like the outreach worker in case example #15 or like the mental health technician in case example #8. She uses activity with the patient/client as a bridge to self-awareness on his part. In this sense her work is intermediate between that of the community worker and that of the mental health technician.

The client was a 35-year-old black male, separated from his wife, who came to the center in February 1971. Apparently he was referred by a doctor and brought by his parents with whom he was staying. He was a college graduate. The extent of withdrawal was unusual, and diagnostically he was thought to have a paranoid schizophrenic reaction. The patient himself had no clearly defined complaint, nor had he any specific ideas about what services he needed, but he did not want to be at home and he did want a job.

The therapist uncovered many indications of overaggressive behavior in the patient's history. He had struck students in the school where he once worked and generally conveyed a kind of suppressed hostility. She thought he needed other channels for the expression of his hostility. She was concerned about his drinking, which she felt was increasing and was something that ought to be discussed. She perceived in the man quite a need for self-expression, which if satisfied might make it possible for him to examine his own feelings with some insight.

Among the interventions employed was encouraging the patient to speak up in the art therapy group about what he was trying to express through his work. He was also encouraged to examine the feelings that came out of the art work. Likewise, he was encouraged to examine relationships within his family. Various techniques were used to elicit some visual representation of his inner conflicts. For example, the therapist asked him to "draw" a kind of table of organization of his life, his family, and the power structure. Having done this, the patient then talked more explicitly about the interrelationships.

Other interventions included group treatment once a week, medication with tranquilizing agents, and participation in the scheduled activities conducted by the center on a regular basis.

The patient completed treatment after some 3 months. During the course of this multipronged therapy he became more self-expressive and had begun work as a jazz musician, an interest he had never totally relinquished. During the following summer, he also held a job with the Department of

Recreation. Currently his exact status is not known, but presumably he is getting along.

Comments. The patient had been referred by a doctor and was brought to the clinic by his parents. The art therapist decided, on the basis of the patient's history, to assist him in seeking more socially acceptable channels for aggressive expression. She felt the patient needed to express himself in order to be able to look at his own feelings. She utilized his productions in art therapy as the vehicle for getting him to explain his feelings to the art therapy group. The work of the art therapist is intermediate between the active doing of the outreach worker and the more passive talking of the mental health technician, and appeared to the Committee to be very similar to the work of a hospital-based activity therapist.

INTERVENTIONS COMPARED

The new interest in community health activities has focused either on the restructuring of the health care delivery system or on the training of additional categories of health workers. Little or no attention has been paid the specific contribution of the community worker to the welfare of his patient/client or the techniques he utilizes in providing the service he delivers.

The Committee explored the work with patient-clients of two categories of community workers: the untrained and the formally trained. As a result of this study, Committee members believe that the patterns and principles behind the worker's interventions with his patient-clients can be delineated. It is our observation that the untrained worker operates in any given instance largely from a base of quite personal experiences with similar problems. He hopes to foster independence by utilizing activity-based techniques. He thereby risks overinvolvement. The trained worker, on the other hand, operates from a base of education and training. He also hopes to foster independence but he utilizes verbal psychotherapy and encourages reflection in his patient to achieve this goal. He risks misjudging the nature of the interaction and the emotional and social response that will be appropriate in the individual situation.

Reference

1. Group for the Advancement of Psychiatry. TOWARD THERAPEUTIC CARE: A GUIDE FOR THOSE WHO WORK WITH THE MENTALLY ILL, 2nd ed. Report No. 77 (New York: GAP, 1970).

3

THE COMMUNITY WORKER: A DESCRIPTION

Community workers make up a heterogeneous group that defies stringent categorization. The background of these workers, their manner of perceiving problems and their fund of knowledge both general and psychiatric often differ from the professionally trained workers', and are directly related to their individual life experiences (see Appendix Tables 3-5).

Background of the community worker

In terms of formal training, the community workers interviewed had varying backgrounds. Some of them were untrained in any formal academic sense, that is, they had never attended a formal academic institution after high school and had received no formal training in the techniques and care of patient-clients under stress. Others had been trained in disciplines unrelated to health or mental health—for example, those trained in art who functioned as art therapists but viewed themselves as community workers. Still others had received undergraduate training in sociology, psychology, or some other liberal arts discipline and functioned, without any additional formal training, in the role of community worker. Thus, the community workers may be viewed along a continuum of training, from those with little or no previous formal training to those having a moderate amount of training in some discipline other than that of mental health.

Another variable of the community worker concerns the previous personal and work experience of the individual. In this connection, the Committee found, as in the case of their training, a wide variation as between one worker and another. Some workers had no previous experience in work situations involving people with health or mental health problems, but they did have extensive personal experience in living and coping in a nonworking setting with people having these problems. Others had little or no previous experience on any level or in any setting with persons having a serious psychiatric or health problem.

Identifying with the client

Perhaps the most significant feature of the experience of the community worker was that it was gained through the process of living, and living in a certain environment. Unlike most professionals who function in an urban community mental health center, most of the community workers lived in the area being served. This made them much more aware of existing realities in the community and enhanced the awareness with which most psychiatric helpers usually begin work on a case. Moreover, the community worker quite often lived in circumstances similar to those of the patient or client he was serving.

Such bonds with patient-clients often can confer special advantages for the worker in relating to, working with, and being accepted by the people of the community he serves. This is only natural, since the community worker is quite likely to have a greater knowledge of the community, its people, and its problems than his more professionally qualified co-workers. Thus he can help the local resident seeking assistance to define his problem more precisely, and he can interpret to the professional worker some features of the presenting problem that might be difficult for the professional to obtain or appreciate. The community worker can interpret to others the culture, the specific ways the patient may be thinking, feeling, speaking, or behaving. He can explain local biases, attitudes, beliefs and social class patterns prevailing in the community. Conversely, he can interpret the professional to clients who may not understand him or are hostile to him for whatever reasons.

If the community worker found a particular problem of health or mental health in one of the families in his neighborhood, the mental health center would be the most likely resource he could call on. In actual practice this varied with the particular community. Presumably, however, this is not necessarily true of workers who have had more formal training and enjoy perhaps higher incomes than their less well-schooled colleagues.

The community workers observed by this committee also identified variously with the community in which the health center was located. Identification was strongest among those who lived in the particular area, and who thereby shared a sense of history and personal involvement aside from their helping stance in the community. This sense of identification was less marked among those living outside the area, who viewed the problems of their client-patients from a greater distance both philosophical and geographical. Unsurprisingly, where the community worker's own reading of the community's sociopolitical realities, problems and solutions paralleled those of the center administrator, he identified more strongly with the center than with his patient-clients.

The racial, ethnic, group identification, and sex of the community worker were by no means unimportant factors in rooting him in the community. For the most part, the workers studied in urban centers by the Committee were black and were women. In areas bordering the suburbs, the community workers were more likely to be white, but here, too, most of them were women. Only in the outreach centers or hot-line centers were men more in evidence. The black community workers explicitly felt they could relate positively to all their patient-clients. Particularly when the patient was also black, there was for him the option of having a black expediter or primary coordinator, who was not readily available in the suburban or outreach centers of the health and mental health system. Another option usually unavailable to the extent needed throughout the health system was that of matching a helper from the same culture as the client—for example, Spanish, Italian or Polish—who understands the culture and the language. The community worker from a "second" culture was more closely identified with the patient/client from the same culture and by his very presence offered an alternative model for imitation.

Manner of perceiving problems

Another important respect in which the community workers varied from one to another was their identification of the patient/client's primary problem, and the central focus of the intervention that should be made. Some community workers felt that the main problems of the needy people in their area were dealing with the social and other support systems that perpetrated a general sense of helplessness among those served. In the eyes of these workers the supporting systems encouraged or actually abetted the poverty of some of those served, while tightening the circle of poverty around others. The thrust of such a community worker's activity would be first directed toward the bureaucratized structure of the social agency and altering its responsiveness to the client; and then educating the client to the role of that agency in his life.

Given this particular point of view, those in the helping stance would tend to deal more with the reality problems of patients brought to the attention of the center than with the mental ills they manifested. This approach offers a balance to the viewpoint that problems develop from within an individual; and more importantly, it creates a working atmosphere that is in keeping with the needs, feelings, and experiences of the patient/client. The patient/client can in this atmosphere view his problems as manageable, and with minimal affront to his self-esteem. Thus he can maintain a high level of motivation and dignity while seeking the help he needs with some confidence in the outcome. This point of view was not shared by all community workers, some taking the position that they must deal primarily with the concern, confusion and difficulties experienced internally by their patient-clients.

Type of knowledge and functions

Generally community workers are persons proficient in the realm of practical activity. Many have had to survive growing up in poverty. They have experienced the discrimination, oppression and resulting hopelessness that so often pervade the neighborhoods in which they work. As a result, they have accumulated a vast array of techniques for survival and growth in situations of enormous stress.

This "know-how of survival" is a vital addition by community workers to current professional practices and attitudes. Such knowledge would enrich the service skills of many professionals, could help many of them develop greater flexibility, efficiency and relevance in the disadvantaged areas of their practice. This know-how could expand the professional capacity to relate to, and work with, people at present unfamiliar with, or previously beyond the reach of, professional assistance. More importantly, however, the "know-how of survival" can be studied, systematized and taught to professional persons needing this input.

Perhaps the most significant way in which community workers described themselves was as that person most closely allied with the patient/client in need of their services. This alliance was made possible by a number of factors:

1—An empathic feeling for what the patient/client was experiencing, including nonverbal nuances.

2—A sense of geographic continuity derived from living in the community during the day while working—but, more importantly, living there after the close of the work day.

3—A feeling that they had themselves lived through experiences similar to those of the clients they were helping, experiences which had given them specific insights into the kind of life stresses experienced by the patient/client and the means by which to manage these stresses.
4—A strong conviction that their previous life experiences had trained them well for the work they were doing and thus had afforded them an understanding of the processes necessary to cope with similar experiences in the lives of others.
5—Greater flexibility and mobility than traditionally trained persons in meeting the patient/client when or where the client so defined the need.
6—Ease of verbal communication in terms of language use and language style.

The community workers also viewed themselves as those in the front line of operations, people who were actively involved in the patient/client's well-being in the sense of aggressively taking charge of the situation. They were dedicated to "doing something" about a problem, not simply discussing it and reporting their reactions to it. Community workers often viewed themselves as patient/client advocates who, when the client was unable to speak for himself, would speak for him. This role also involved their helping the client to negotiate successfully the multiple systems that determine the level and quality of patient care. These systems comprise those particularly related to the patient, his family, and their interpersonal relationships, as well as those involving the professional network of welfare, mental health, general health and supporting social structures.

Moreover, many of the community workers interviewed saw themselves as the expediter, the link or liaison between the professional and the client when difficulties in communication arise. Quite often these community workers commented on the failure of professional persons to understand the particular requests or the particular point of view held by the client. Here the community worker acts as a bridge between the recipient of services and the professional provider, between the resident of the community and community resources. He resides at the port of entry into the service system and assumes the responsibility of helping the resident define his problem and of determining the specific service required to meet it.

The community worker interprets to the patient/client the services and programs of the agency; likewise he may interpret the specific needs of his client, his manner and behavior, his anxieties and expectations, to the agency, so that in turn the agency may gear its services to the individual needs of the client. In this role the community worker may act as translator, interpreter, negotiator, legal aide, educator and model.

The community worker can serve the client as educator and instructor. He can inform the client of the resources available to him, his rights and responsibilities, and the best way to go about obtaining the services he may need. He can teach the client how best to approach certain agencies and professionals, how to speak to them, impress them, and utilize them.

Other advantages stemming from the life style and knowledge of the community worker become evident in agency efforts to reach the extremely disadvantaged. The limits of professionals in working with such people as school dropouts, delinquents, drug addicts and militant groups are well documented. These limitations are aggravated by the fact that services either have been inadequate or have been so organized and operated as to restrict severely their use by these people. Since the community worker himself has generally been recruited from a population also hard to reach, he is in a position to enter into the community, gain and maintain contact with those alienated from the common sources of service. He is able to complement and extend professional services and to bring about the adjustments necessary to keep programs and professionals interested and involved.

In general, an accurate description of the community

worker essentially requires recognition of the diversity of individuals functioning in this role. Diversity characterizes every basic feature of the person and the job: (1) previous formal training, (2) previous life and work experience, (3) identification with racial and ethnic groups served, (4) concept of the fundamental problems that must be addressed and how one deals with those problems, (5) the alliance or association perceived with the particular patient/client, and (6) the concern as an active involved helper in the front line of operations.

4

CONSIDERATIONS IN TRAINING THE COMMUNITY WORKER

TRAINING PROGRAMS

To bring this new dimension of health care service personified in the community worker to its optimum potential, we cannot depend on job-oriented supervision, consultation, and hit-or-miss inservice training programs. The plight of the community worker, his need for useful credentials, and the dilemma of those entrusted with his further training are revealed in the statement which follows:[1]

> I am the Director of Outreach for a neighborhood health center. I am a combination administrator, supervisor, and social worker. Yet I have had little formal training and no credentials. Paraprofessionals have always had obstacles to face. My own experiences provide a good basis for an analysis of the role of professionals and paraprofessionals in the health field today. As I advanced in my own field, I began to discover many subtleties in the attitudes of professionals which indicated to me that I was not considered as being on the same or even a different level as they. The credentialed professional does not know how to accept me. His terms used to identify me hide an implicit professional racism: "paraprofessional," "subprofessional," "nonprofessional," and so on. He earns far more money and holds decision-making power. The reason is obvious to all of us; he holds a degree and I do not.
>
> Whatever the reasons that account for his having received the education rather than me, those who work in the health and health-related fields today must be ready to deal with

> and to utilize effectively the immense manpower available. We all hear of the manpower shortage, but what of the huge number of noncredentialed people whose vast life experiences may have served as training for careers in human services? I serve patients who come to the health center from the neighborhood in which I live. I am involved in their lives and I always have been. Because of my experiences, I may be able to perform more significant and far-reaching human services for these patients than the physician himself, in spite of his formal education.
>
> Yet as I become more involved in decision making within the system, I must train myself to be constantly aware, emotionally and intellectually, that the system itself must be negotiated with for the patient's benefit; this is my job. At times I must convince my fellow workers that this is my true concern, rather than a search for personal power, and I must keep myself aware of [this] as well. The professional must be willing, through some kind of ongoing dialogue and even inservice training for staff, to accept an untrained (from his point of view) and noncredentialed person as a member of the primary care team. It is clear that we must reach the people who are our pateints. The professional is a technician—it is most often the paraprofessional who is best equipped to provide the human service, drawing on the resources of the professional. There must be a concerted effort to build a structure within which staff can perform with a mutual bond of respect and recognition, or human services cannot be delivered. The training that must be provided is not for the paraprofessional alone. He must cease trying to imitate and emulate the professional. He must use his own skills.

Much has been published about the community mental health worker and similar categories of workers, but only a small number of these publications focus on training and education. Although unique programs are described that appear to have merit, prevalent training patterns are not discernible. In fact, formal training may be relegated to a position of minor importance, with the emphasis on utilizing those qualities and resources of community mental health workers that derive from their personal and social background.

The needs of both the client population served and the service organization are not always clearly differentiated or reflected in training programs. Since the Committee was unable to perceive a consistent pattern in the training programs studied, our comments will in many instances be generalizations from a diverse range of programs either noted or described in the literature. While the need for an extensive description of training goals and standards is imperative, it is beyond the scope of this report.

Community workers are categorized in many ways. Such a diversity of education and experience prevails among them that one of the first issues to be addressed is that of their identity vis à vis the traditional professionals with whom they are associated in their work. As has been noted, community workers are a heterogeneous group and are referred to by many titles. They are frequently categorized, not with regard to the tasks they perform, but by characteristics and qualities they have in common, such as "indigenous." Apparently there is a tendency on the part of these workers to perceive themselves as different from others in their community, even though one of their major assets would seem to be their close relationship with the community they serve.

In this connection, the Kentucky Mental Health Manpower Commission[2] employed a useful classification of job characteristics for "middle level" mental health workers. The Commission outlines three basic types: Type I is the Community Mental Health Aide. Workers in this group function as client agents and advocates in an outreach case-finding and preventive service. Type II is the Community Mental Health Technician, who works as a therapeutic agent providing professional help. Type III, the Community Mental Health Representative, functions as a systems agent and as liaison with other agencies and services.

Committee members endorse the development of programs which (1) structure the training of the worker, (2) clearly define how his talents are to be utilized, and (3) provide a means for evaluating his effectiveness. There is probably a high risk of chaos in health delivery systems where multidisciplinary teams at all levels of sophistication work together without clearly delineated functional responsibilities.

In some instances, the worker may elect, after gaining training and experience, to enter one of the more traditional professional groups. There is a need on the part of the workers for appropriate recognition of their skills, and where they are not recognized, competitive struggles with professionals may frequently ensue. There are practical reasons for their wish to be considered as a group with rights equivalent to those of professionals. Their interests, responsibilities and work assignments may be similar to those of professionals in the same organization. It seems realistic to allow workers to progress up an organizational ladder rather than to lock them into a blind alley. This need for upward mobility has been recognized in various agencies, and occasionally groups have been encouraged to form unions or other group associations with their peers. For all practical purposes, of course, these organizations are not often found.

Riessman[3] has stressed the importance of organization, as well as the commitment of the worker to the community. With the support of his agency and teachers, the community worker can establish new identifications without compromising his valuable ties in the community. If this can be accomplished for the majority of community workers, not only will they continue to contribute what they do best in the system of health care, but they will also be fulfilling their own educational and training needs.

Recent consumer pressure for more comprehensive mental health care has called our attention to the desirability of involving many more care providers in the delivery system. Although they realize the desirability of expanding their services, traditional professional groups are sometimes reluctant to acknowledge the value or understand the nature of the services offered by the "new" mental health worker. It should be apparent that simply by training more of the same types of professionals we will not necessarily be in position to meet the needs of the people, yet "closed shop" and "sacred turf" attitudes too often persist. Moreover it has been demonstrated that with the proper support, certain key categories in the community service network are able to and do perform many services previously unmet by the more traditional delivery systems, or by professionals. In this situation the community worker adds significantly to the resources available for meeting patient/client needs.

Because of the variety of categories for mental health workers, it is not surprising to find many different kinds of training programs evolving as the growing need for them comes to the surface. In reviewing the literature and from communications with some of those responsible for supervising community workers, one finds a wide range of standards and training curricula prevailing. By and large, these apply to personnel who do not belong to one of the traditional professions. They may or may not be high school graduates. They usually have some common tie with the persons served. For instance, they may be ex-addicts, ex-prison inmates, school dropouts, or exceptional members of some disadvantaged minority. They have in common the desire to provide more effective care for the hard-to-reach members of the community.

Undoubtedly many complex factors enter into the motivations of those going the paraprofessional route. In many instances it would seem that these paraprofessionals have been unable to obtain a compatible job-oriented education for many reasons—they may have been economically disadvantaged; may not have decided their career goals early enough; early educational experiences may have been so diffuse or inadequate that it was not possible to sustain an interest in continuing their education; in some cases family needs may have precluded development of a career via full-time scholastic training. At any rate, there appear to be as many complex reasons why these workers did not take the traditional professional path as there are reasons why they subsequently became interested in this sort of work.

It should be useful to differentiate training programs which are remedial in content from those geared to the specific activities in which the trainees are involved. This, in fact, may disclose the need for a major effort on the part of program planners to define more clearly the role and function of the various professionals also serving in the agency, since there is both overlap and failure to specify limits in these areas so far as this committee has been able to determine.

The mental health worker has training and educational needs that are common to all of us in the field. In part, this training can be viewed as personally useful and in part as adding to a professional understanding and technical equipment in the prosecution of health care activities. In the latter area, one solution has attempted to provide an educational program in which both professionals and nonprofessionals participate together. Although this grouping runs counter to tradition, there is something to be said for it in that each trainee group has much to contribute to the other. Thus, both professionals and nonprofessionals may come away from such a training experience with a more accurate understanding of the problems encountered in the delivery of caretaking services.[4]

Most service agencies recognize that the indigenous worker has unique skills and talents for understanding and working with people who have practical, personal and social problems. Here a psychosocial orientation appears to be more valued than the traditional medical model. The scope of formal training requirements ranges from none at all to several years. Most service organizations utilizing such personnel, however, do require continuing on-the-job training as a minimum requirement for the job. Most allow the training and the job to proceed concurrently even when the training is quite extensive—for example, in a community college. In some of these colleges an associate degree may be obtained, with the possibility that graduates may return later for enrollment in an academic program. In many cases, training is provided chiefly to foster the development of skills and permit progression up the line in a graduated system of classified nonprofessional positions.

Frequently the worker trainee is one who has already demonstrated skills in working with people, and the training program is designed to increase his understanding of interpersonal relationships and the complexities of human communication. In the process of surveying what has been written about the training of workers, Committee members have found that it is possible in a general way to determine who is being trained. Some notion of content can also be derived. The format of training programs is variable. Often, the training program correlates with the job experience and involves individual supervision and small-group experience. Although a didactic approach may be used, this does not seem to be the predominant mode. The training curriculum resembles that for the mental health clinician more than a typical college program, but utilizes both educational styles.

Some such programs deal specifically with the development of interpersonal skills and an understanding of human relationships; others are designed along more general educational lines. Representative of the more organized curricula, Lynch and Gardner[5] include a number of general headings in an outline of one curriculum. This curriculum utilizes classroom discussion and sensitivity groups as well as didactic material addressing relevant problems like language skills, health care and health patterns, black identity, social issues, psychological development, psychiatric interviewing, and psychopathology. Danzig[6] includes courses in literature, writing, music, mathematics, visual arts, American Civilization and the Contemporary World. Others are offered under titles like Human Growth and Development, Principles of Sociology, Social Problems and Agency Resources, Sociology of the Family, Cultural and Ethnic Minority Groups, and Cultural Anthropology. The behavioral sciences are broadly represented.

A representative curriculum typically focuses on helping the trainee to understand human development and the varied social and cultural elements that are a part of the human scene. In addition to familiarizing the student with traditional clinical entities, courses are designed to increase the student's understanding of the family and of social disorders.

How training programs are evaluated and rewarded is not clear to the Committee. Obviously, if a trainee earns a college degree, he also earns some measure of official sanction, but this is not the situation in many agencies. Some have sought to define the qualities desired in terms that can be measured with psychological tests. Others have correlated job classification with the completion of training programs. In general, however, training programs seem to be aimed at better equipping the worker for his job, and in a sense are pragmatically oriented in favor of the "consumer" and the employer. That this is important to all would be generally accepted. It therefore follows that it would be useful if it could be more explicitly spelled out just where community workers fit into the delivery of mental health care and exactly how their contributions may be effectively evaluated. Currently some agencies are attempting to address this problem.

Finally, there is no clear-cut system of formal recognition and reward analogous to that seen in a typical professional degree program. Yet establishing guidelines for training and defining standards for training goals would seem to favor the achievement of a stronger and more satisfying identity by these new mental health workers as they complete training curricula based on them. Many experimental programs are under way. But there seems to be a need for more coordinated efforts in the development of programs defining standards and goals which not only foster personal development but also provide many levels of function. These programs should provide trainees with formal recognition and rewards.

PROFESSIONAL BACKUP, SUPERVISION AND CONSULTATION

Just as there are many names for the community worker, there are many definitions of what it is these workers do. It follows that the answers are just as varied to the question what it is they should be taught to do and should be able to do. It would also appear that how the professionals relate to this new category of worker in terms of supervision and consultation would quite naturally reveal great variety and complexity. In all eleven of the outreach programs that members of our committee visited, supervision and consultation for the community workers from their professional colleagues was indicated to be available, but this situation raised more questions than it answered. For example, how do we interpret what is meant by "available" as compared to being "available and used," or as compared to being "available and well used"?

The real goals of the professionals involved side by side with the community workers and *their* goals are quite relevant to the questions that must be answered. The indigenous worker who really wants to be left alone to "do his thing" in relationship to his clients is very different from the individual who has an eye on a spot within one of the professional disciplines and regards himself as being upwardly mobile in the system.

Another question: Is the "available" supervision and consultation really usable, or is it merely an attempt to transfer professional expertise from one area of activity and to use it as the ongoing education of the neighborhood worker? When one examines a great variety of these training programs—the great diversity of short- and long-term education and training courses to which prospective and current community workers have been subjected, it is difficult to ream out a common core of what they need to know and what constitutes their role. What a community worker does, certainly, is to provide human service. On the other hand, his role is certainly not limited to a fragment of expertise from one of the already existing professions in the service network. The how and the where of this human service has some degree of uniqueness even though it—like the human service provided by the traditional professionals in mental health services—has at its center the interpersonal relationship between the service worker and the recipient of the service. And like the goal of the traditional mental health professionals, the goal of the community worker is to bring about constructive change in the person and the situation of the recipient.

The indigenous community advocate. In one of the neighborhood action programs observed by Committee members, the community workers, who are black, are indigenous to the catchment area. They all have a high school education or less, plus some noncredit, dead-end training courses. These workers consider themselves community advocates and tend to feel exploited, with little or no recognition accorded them for their special skills. They feel that the really valued individuals in the project are those who hold degrees. It is unclear what the agency's statement that supervision is available from staff social workers really means. It may not be so unclear that there is supervisory influence from their peers, but it is unclear just how far the stated availability of psychiatric consultation really goes. The specific complaint voiced by some was that social work supervision was not formal enough and that evaluations of their efforts were infrequent. On the other hand, it was very clear to this committee that these workers get a great deal of satisfaction out of working with their psychiatric consultant at the level of case presentations and case discussions.

One of the workers interviewed was uncomfortable with a role shift in which she was involved, from that of a home management specialist to that of a community worker, which in the eyes of the neighborhood workers is more like the role of a social worker. An examination of the field reports reveals a not too close correlation between the skills of this indigenous worker advocate and the capacities of the mental health workers in the program who hold degrees which might be utilized to add to this worker's abilities through supervision of her work and consultation with her. It would also appear that the worker herself was not fully satisfied that she enjoyed any real backup from the more classically trained members of the mental health team.

The bilingual factor. In another neighborhood program operating from a planning and service center, the worker interviewed was indigenous to the area and also to the particular clientele being served, being Puerto Rican by birth, and bilingual. This woman is a high school graduate and as an advocate within the community functions mainly on her knowledge of the community and of the nature of the particular problems of the clients. In this situation, she had direct and frequent access to the support and supervision of the director of the center and in addition had excellent working relationships with the clinical consultants in related agencies, from whom she appears to have frequently and advantageously sought consultation or supervision. In this situation the worker evidenced little concern about her lack of a college degree and expressed not a little comfort in the fact that her backup support was coming from a staff some of whose consulting members were also Puerto Rican.

Self-realization. A drop-in center for addicts appeared to be a very different kind of outreach project compared to the other neighborhood centers visited. The community workers are white and many of them are former drug users. This is a self-organized group in no way a health facility by its own definitions, although the organization has a great many informal contacts with health agencies, including private psychiatric hospitals. The whole program is group meeting-oriented, and there is little use for the usual consultations or supervision other than that provided by one consultant, who sits in on the group meetings on a scheduled basis. The community workers at this center are mostly college graduates, and the focus on their part as well as the clients' is "self-realization."

Another outreach program conducted from a neighborhood service center is referred to as a "supermarket of services." This program utilizes indigenous black workers who have a high school education. Their functions are very broad and they perceive themselves as involved community organizers. Here again, it is very difficult for the Committee to spell out the implications of these workers' statements that there is little supervision but they could use more, because they obviously place a high value on their independent function and their ready access to each other for support. In this organization, consultation is considered available but is very little used.

Former aides. In an outreach project serving children and youth, which functions within a city-county health department, there is yet another pattern. The neighborhood workers are black and indigenous, with usually a high school education, but they are all former psychiatric hospital aides. They enjoy the regular supervision of a social worker and a pediatrician and also have access to professional consultation with other specialists, among them a public health nurse and a psychiatrist. This pattern would appear to be very like the usual pattern of supervision to be found in an inpatient psychiatric program.

Yet another community health project offers its community workers supervision and consultation very much like that provided the workers in the youth project. Here the neighborhood workers are also indigenous to the area and are black. Likewise they are high school-educated and come to their jobs after several years of supervised aide work in either a private or a public psychiatric hospital. They work with a much wider latitude than that enjoyed as psychiatric aides, but they are backed up by continuous supervision and by consultation with the project social worker. Regular psychiatric consultation is also assigned.

Collaboration and consultation. A comprehensive community mental health center associated with a university department of psychiatry and an OEO program offers its workers other dimensions of backup and development. The neighborhood worker is a social worker with a master's degree who functions independently but works very closely with all other involved disciplines through consultation and collaboration and in particular with one psychologist as a peer.

A state-wide emergency service and crisis intervention clinic, which is a component of a community mental health center, utilizes a white indigenous neighborhood worker who considers himself a generalist in mental health because of his associate arts degree. He works under supervision as a sort of junior-grade diagnostician and reality-oriented short-term therapist. His backup consists of half an hour a week of psychiatric consultation and one weekly staff conference of 2 hours' duration.

The day center of one health department program, which is to be a unit of a mental health center, departs completely from the spectrum of backup and consultative patterns already discussed. The community worker is white and not indigenous to the area. She performs the outreach function of integrating patients served by the organization into the community rather than the reverse. She is able to do this by utilizing a high degree of skill developed in the course of obtaining her A.B. degree in art. Three 1-hour case conferences a week, psychological consultation, and a whole team for backup give her supervisory and consultative support.

Clinical "togetherness." Another large metropolitan area has four mental health centers operating in a still different pattern. These community workers at the centers may or may not be indigenous. They are assigned to clinical teams and there is a great effort to achieve role diffusion and offer variety in clinical assignments. There appeared to be a great deal of clinical togetherness in these teams, the training of whose members ranges all the way from completely unskilled to classically trained, multidegreed mental health workers. While in one sense there is no supervision, a high level of clinical togetherness and mutual support is maintained for the neighborhood workers who operate out of these four centers.

Degree-oriented workers. At another mental health center, the white neighborhood worker interviewed was indigenous to the area. He had a high school diploma and while working was taking a counseling curriculum at a local college. The function of this worker was that of a bridge between the professional providing the mental health services and the residents of the catchment area, by way of setting up initial contacts and also by organizing group sessions. This worker was supervised regularly by a child psychiatrist and a social worker. However, she was burdened with the problem attendant upon being directed toward a degree while at the same time feeling annoyance at having to get her written work countersigned by a professional.

Comment. The eleven different programs visited and reviewed revealed a wide variety of types of consultation, supervision and backup afforded an equally wide variety of community workers. Many of the working relationships observed between the neighborhood workers and their professional backup have evolved out of the capacities and limitations of the individuals on the team, rather than from any thought-out blending of skills and functions based on job descriptions.

This was probably unavoidable at the time of planning, when there were no job descriptions available to make possible an assessment of how the backup professional could supervise and/or consult with the worker in meeting goals and assignments as yet unclear.

In some of the programs examined, the barrier between the community workers and the backup professional seemed formidable. The workers felt misunderstood and unappreciated, while the backup team felt they had made themselves available but were not being used, even though this might in part be due to ignorance of the goals of the support being offered. Consultation and supervision seemed least variable in agencies where attempts to inform the worker better and render him better able to operate as a neighborhood worker were reinforced by attempts to develop him into a junior-grade professional.

It also became clear that the more nearly the community worker could identify with the backup professional—by previous experience (former aide), by previous education (mental health degree or associate or college degree), by concurrent college attendance, or by working in a situation of planned role diffusion—the less apparent the status difference between the worker and the classical mental health professional. In a relative sense, however, this greater closeness between the community worker and the professionals on the service team was achieved at community expense, for there appeared to be less outreach in the function of the workers, who were less available to the members of the community.

The task involved in providing the community worker with the professional backup he needs through supervision and consultation must thus be approached with several critical factors in mind. First, his functions must be defined, giving primary importance to his indigenous status, the values of which should not be lost in the delivery of services. Second, he must be appropriately remunerated for services rendered at the same time that he is given the backup and support he needs in order to carry out his neighborhood functions properly. The end product would be a community worker so secure in his job description and his functions that he could utilize the consultation and supervision of a full spectrum of professional disciplines without demeaning his own position, without jealousy for the academic degrees of the professionals with whom he works on the one hand or feelings of second-class citizenship on the other. Only as he works in this interpersonal way, with his goal the goal of all, can he provide service to the client-patients out of which constructive change can come.

References

1. Shirley Wigfall & Anna H. Mace. A Paraprofessional Speaks, *Sandoz Psychiatric Spectator* (an Ortho Summary) Vol 8, No. 4 (1972) abstract.
2. Community Mental Health Workers. Project Reports (Louisville, Ky: Kentucky Mental Health Manpower Commission, 1971).
3. Frank Riessman. Strategies and Suggestions for Training Nonprofessionals, *Community Mental Health Journal* 3, 2 (Summer 1967): 103-110.
4. Sheldon K. Schiff. Training the Professional, *University of Chicago Magazine* 62, 4 (1970).
5. Mary Lynch & Elmer Gardner. Some Issues Raised in the Training of Paraprofessionals as Clinic Therapists, *American Journal of Psychiatry* 126, 10 (1970): 1473-1480.
6. Martin E. Danzig. Education of the Community Mental Health Assistant: Dovetailing Theory with Practice, *Mental Hygiene* 54, 3 (July 1970): 357-363.

5

INFLUENCE OF THE ORGANIZATION ON DELIVERY OF SERVICE

Community-based facilities like mental health centers, neighborhood health centers and multiservice centers have been developed under differing auspices—some public, some private. Some were started by providers, some by consumers. Some are located in general health facilities, some in specialized mental health settings, still others in social agencies. This pluralistic origin has created widely differing service models.

Given good leadership, adequate funding, and no little determination, it may be possible to carry out a well-defined program regardless of the organizational setting. Realistically, however, programs at variance with the organizational context in which they operate seldom reach the level of success. For one thing, the expenditure of effort in opposing organizational forces is too costly. Inevitably, constraints imposed by the organization exert an impact on the individual worker and influence his activities in his role as a caregiver.

Several organizational phenomena may influence the kind and quality of services that can be rendered by the individual worker—the organization's system of formal job classification, its governing body, the basis of funding, its formally stated purposes, underlying treatment philosophy, and interaction with the community.

Formal classification

Patterns of care will differ widely among the organizations providing it. A hospital, a free-standing outpatient facility, a social agency, or an interested citizens' group will inevitably develop a pattern of care differing sharply from the patterns of the others. Control of all health service organizations is becoming increasingly more stringent. Regulations may be enforced by many authorities in the form of licensure, governmental safety requirements, accreditation standards of voluntary accrediting agencies, governmental requirements for funding, the demands of private third-party payers, the mechanism of comprehensive health planning agencies, and by many other mechanisms. Thus a specific service provided by a worker in a hospital would be subjected to drastically different standards and requirements than the identical service rendered by a worker in a free-standing outpatient facility.

In addition to requirements imposed by outside agencies, the professional groups working in the service setting have significant influence. For example, in a hospital all treatment services must be rendered under the supervision of a physician who is legally responsible for the actions of every individual performing a service under his direction, and patterns of care will therefore by heavily influenced by the medical model. The orientation of caregivers in a nonmedical setting would likely have a different character.

Case example #1. Consider the case of the 14-year-old girl who telephoned a drop-in clinic because she was depressed, confused and concerned about her use of drugs. She was offered an opportunity to talk things over. Because her parents were critical of the life style of the personnel at the drop-in clinic, she was assured that her parents would not be informed of the clinic's involvement. A few days later when she called saying that she had slashed her wrists, a worker went to the home and gave first aid. It was only when she came to the drop-in clinic after running away from home that the worker insisted she tell her parents what was going on. (See also Section 1, Case example #1.)

In responding to the girl's plea for help, a worker in a hospital would have been providing a medical service and could not have done so without the full knowledge and permission of the child's parents. The rendering of first aid, even for a minor injury, would have been unthinkable without recourse to consultation with a health professional. The relatively unstructured basis for offering help to a youngster who might be considered a suicidal risk and the lack of any formalized treatment plan would not have been acceptable in a hospital-sponsored service.

Arguments can be mustered favoring the approach ordinarily used in either setting. The issue is not which is the superior approach. Rather the point being emphasized is that the standards, requirements, and attitudes of the facility have a major influence on the worker's options for intervention.

Characteristics of the governing body

In any organization or institution, some group or individual has the final responsibility and authority. In the voluntary health institutions this has commonly been a board established under appropriate local, state, and sometimes federal laws. Governmental institutions have usually been controlled by some bureaucratic entity such as a commission, a board, or an administration set up by an elected governing body and thus ultimately responsible to the voters.

Such governing bodies have been dimly perceived in organizations and have often attended primarily to the management of finances and property, while showing little interest and undertaking little activity in the area of program content. There have been notable exceptions and within recent years there has been a growing emphasis on involving the consumer and making the composition of the governing body more broadly representative of the population served.

Likewise governing bodies are increasingly taking a direct interest in program content and the manner in which services are provided. Since the governing body controls the resources, it can exert a decisive influence on what occurs in any setting. The individual health care worker will seldom have any direct communication with the governing body and thus is dependent upon management-inspired communications that come down "through channels" with all the misinterpretations and distortions that may be added on the way. Nevertheless, he is influenced by what he believes to be the policies of the governing body and he certainly will be affected by the decisions made regarding the allocation of resources.

For example, one of the centers visited was for all practical purposes controlled by the County Health Officer, who in turn was accountable to the County Council. It was believed that the County Health Officer, and presumably the City Council, preferred that mental health issues be subsumed under the rubric of total health care. The center was not permitted to use nonprofessionals in any meaningful way to provide care; the caregivers were a part-time psychiatrist, a social worker, and a part-time nurse. Consequently, the services provided were traditional in type and limited in nature, consisting primarily of weekly individual psychotherapy and some follow-up of discharged state hospital patients for maintenance drug therapy.

Although the Center had been open for a few years, it was not felt to be a part of the community. Resistance and suspicion were expressed about the location of the center in the community, with some grumbling about the parking problems. Inaccessibility of services to those in lower socioeconomic brackets persisted. Some professionals had advocated a more vigorous approach to the community but the assumptions made about the County Health Officer's attitude and the limited support from the County Council determined the types of workers employed and pushed the professionals in the direction of providing services that would be inconspicuous and noncontroversial.

Contrast this situation with that prevailing in a mental

health center of a large urban area whose president characterized it as "an umbrella agency" with the immediate goals of (1) strengthening residents' participation in health center planning and program, and (2) increasing community support that would enable the center to expand. The Association's roster included informed professionals, members of the clergy, civic leaders, and concerned residents.

Newspaper articles quoting the governing board leaders described the center as enjoying an "informal, noninstitutional approach," as "trying to tumble outdated barriers," and as "taking involved and activist approaches to community health, veering sharply from the detached professionalism of medicine in past decades."

One worker in this center viewed herself as a "grass roots person" able to bridge the gap between team professionals and residents of the community. She was active in a street counselor project that involved socializing with the teenagers and young adults at night in the town square and nearby cafes. She knew she would be supported in responding to the extraordinary, even if this meant agreeing "to come quickly at 2:00 a.m. and rap for several hours." The organizational setting clearly pushed her toward interventions that she and the leadership of the center considered relevant.

Source of funding

The funding of programs has always had a significant impact on content because the resources available limit the scope of any program. But in recent years those responsible for paying the bill have become far more direct in their control. With 40 percent of the nation's health care paid for by government, and most of the rest through private insurance, the potential for using the funding mechanism to control services has become a reality. When services are paid for on a fee basis, the shape of a program and the activities of the health worker can be controlled by the schedule of benefits. For programs that get their funding through government appropriation or some type of grant, the workers' interventions can be decisively influenced by fear of compromising continued financial support.

For example, an emergency service and crisis clinic for a catchment area housing approximately 160,000 residents was funded through a state grant administered at the county level. As originally conceptualized, the main thrust of the program was (1) to provide emergency services 24 hours a day for all residents of the catchment, (2) to offer crisis intervention with short-term treatment, and (3) to direct patients toward appropriate longer-term treatment resources in the community. It was planned that the emphasis would be on achieving therapeutic results rather than on processing people simply to make an expedient disposition of cases handled.

As the program got under way, an increasing number of requests came from the medical officer at the county jail, which happened to be located within the catchment area but served the entire county population of over 600,000. While some of these requests were suited to the services of the clinic (emergency and crisis intervention), many were simply for assistance in the disposition of prisoners by such measures as providing a second physician's certificate for involuntary commitment.

As time went by, an effort was even made to place responsibility on the crisis program for preventing the incarceration of any individual thought to have a psychiatric disorder. Although supported by the clinic staff, this objective was enormous in scope, requiring as it did changes in the state hospital system, modification of the judicial system, and the development of new treatment resources.

Nevertheless, the staff was not long in assessing the influence the judiciary could exert on the political process, and realized that the future of the crisis program might be dependent upon their response to the demands of the county jail. The workers felt a strong pressure to respond to referrals from the jail by meeting the demand for rapid disposition of cases, with less emphasis on therapeutic intervention.

Purposes of the organization

Outreach workers are employed in many organizations that do not have health care as their primary purpose. In consequence, the outreach worker often sees himself as working within a much broader context, giving help on financial matters, legal questions, educational problems, and a miscellany of common personal problems, while the health care professional tends to limit the range of his activities toward the giving of health care.

When an outreach worker works within an organization that does have health care as its primary purpose, he is apt to feel some pressure to narrow the definition of his services in consonance with the stated purpose of the organization. Even within an organization limited to health care, the purpose is sometimes ambiguous. Are the many federal and state drug abuse programs primarily intended to provide a health service to addicts, or are they primarily directed toward crime prevention by diminishing the need of the addict to maintain his drug habit by stealing?

Case example #5. The activities of one community worker in helping a married couple may well have been influenced by the purposes of the organization which employed her—a multiservice agency set up to provide a "supermarket of needed services." (See also Section 1, Case example #5, preceding.) Under this program the outreach worker attempted to respond to the needs of the client by utilizing and directing the client to a wide range of potential services, among them legal aid, family services, education, recreation, welfare, food and nutrition, health services, vocational rehabilitation, and still others.

This community worker had discovered the couple, who

were both alcoholic, in going from door to door in the community. The wife was crippled and the husband unemployed. The worker got them welfare vouchers for food and rent. She helped the wife to get better clothing, visit a beautician, and straighten up the house. The husband was assisted, through vocational rehabilitation, in getting a job as a truck driver. The worker, who visited this couple many times, was gratified to find that they had both stopped drinking even though she had not taken definitive action about their alcoholism and despite their failure to follow up on her suggestion that they go to an alcoholism information center for help.

Just as the worker's efforts seemed to be crowned by success, the couple began drinking again, returning to their old pattern of living, and completely rejected the worker. Surprised, bewildered and hurt by this development, she considers the case one of her worst failures. In retrospect she felt that she had had little understanding of the problems of the alcoholic and had thus failed to concentrate her further efforts on this problem. The many supportive activities she provided, while of great value, failed to touch the core problem.

The multipurpose orientation of the organization probably influenced this worker toward a multifaceted supportive approach, where a worker from an organization oriented toward mental health, and particularly alcoholism services, undoubtedly would have approached the couple with an emphasis on treating the alcoholism, and with possibly a different outcome.

Philosophy of the treatment setting

The specific treatment philosophy of a particular facility is influenced in varying degree by the governing board, the type of facility, and the professional orientation of the key personnel. While to a great extent treatment philosophy may be shaped by program directors, it must be reinforced by the framework within which it is carried out. For example, professionals who subscribe to the five basic services of a community mental health center (inpatient, outpatient, partial hospitalization, emergency and crisis intervention, and consultative and educational services) will be attracted to community mental health centers and will, in their program planning, incorporate their particular interpretation of this philosophy.

These general principles will be amplified by more specific philosophies—as, for example, the team approach versus the individual approach; brief crisis-oriented intervention versus long-term therapies; utilization of indigenous workers as opposed to the more highly trained professionals, and so on. Though stated as polar opposites, there will be a range of treatment philosophies within any setting, with the model somewhere along the continuum of care. Such treatment philosophies may be explicitly spelled out but often they are communicated through conferences, supervision of workers, and the role models provided by leaders of the program.

For example, one center in a metropolitan area emphasized a team approach in which the basic question to be answered at the outset is, "What is this *customer* asking for?" Further emphasis was placed on the social issues of the patients' lives and on the manner in which these problems are met by the community. Although some team members might have an individual psychological orientation, the prevailing viewpoint concerned the effect of the broader psychosocial ills on patient/client interaction. Those seeking help were seen more in the context of their total living systems than in terms of their intrapsychic problems.

These treatment philosophies pushed individual workers of the center in the direction of seeking practical solutions for reality problems rather than applying individual therapeutic techniques. Even the approach to specific symptoms was one of trying to "cool them down" so that the patient could accommodate to changes in the environmental system and accept them. There tended to be a similarity in the tasks carried out by the various members of the team, with the more highly trained professionals handling those situations where the client demanded a professional, or where their professional status was an asset, as, for example, in dealing with other professionals.

Response to the population served

Any service system gets a feedback from the population served. In more sophisticated programs special evaluation procedures may be utilized to insure a continuing influence on the service system based on the response of patients being treated. Even without such formalized evaluative systems and plans for consumer participation, the worker will be influenced by the people with whom he interacts to serve.

An illustration of this effect on a community worker can be seen in an outreach multiservice agency located in a large city. The career of the worker interviewed began somewhat by accident after she had noticed that many professionals who did not speak Spanish were unable to communicate successfully with the many Spanish-speaking clients and patients served by this center. Because she had a good command of English as well as Spanish, having grown up in Puerto Rico, she felt she could bridge this gap. She readily grasped the general approach to the health needs of the people in her area, but because of her past experience developed a deep sympathy with the struggle of the newly arrived Puerto Rican. Thus she usually conceptualized the problems of those seeking help in terms of their conflicts and struggles to survive on the mainland with its new values and new demands.

Case example #13. This worker described her work with a 17-year-old unmarried Puerto Rican male accused of inflicting cigarette burns on his 1-year-old nephew (see Section 1, Case example #13, preceding). The family perceived this as an emergency situation possibly best solved by arranging for the boy's return to Puerto Rico. An organic basis for his behavior was suggested by a history of severe head trauma with skull fracture and treatment with anticonvulsive medication. The patient seemed distressed and ready to accept the solution of his problems by returning to Puerto Rico.

Because of her particular sensitivity to the needs of this cultural group, the worker focused on the problems the patient was having in adjusting to his new environment. She perceived the problem as being more one of an adjustment reaction than one caused by organic pathology or intrapsychic disorder. In consequence, she directed her efforts toward helping the family provide a setting and living conditions that would enhance the patient's self-esteem while she looked for tangible ways by which he could be more successfully adjusted to life in the United States. As her attempts were successful, his symptoms abated.

In many ways the interventions of this agency were especially designed to meet the needs of the Spanish-speaking resident population. For example, the agency's concern about the problems in the city school system, where the Spanish-speaking children were scorned by both children and teachers for not knowing English, prompted direct action. They forced the school system to establish bilingual classes and to be more accepting of the various cultural differences between the American and the Spanish-speaking pupils. The agency sponsored community events—for one event preparing a float for the San Juan Day parade at the State House so that the youngsters and adults of the Spanish-speaking residents could take pride in their background rather than experience their differences as inadequacies that were a cause for shame. Thus, the program within this health center and the specific interventions of the workers took on a special character because of the population served.

Comment

In our study of the care-giving activities of individual workers, Committee members became aware that these could be understood only in relation to the context in which they were provided. We did not try to study or analyze the organizational systems *per se*. Rather we sought to identify some of the major means by which the organizational setting influences the services provided, and to draw attention to the need to take this influence into consideration in any assessment of the care-giving services provided by the community workers.

6

CURRENT AND FUTURE ISSUES

Earlier in this report, the Committee pointed out that its members are practitioners quite aware of the therapeutic procedures, practices and interventions used in mental hospitals, psychiatric wards, and outpatient clinics. In the newer community health and mental health facilities visited, the roles and functions of psychiatrists, nurses, psychologists and social workers were similar, though greatly influenced by the community context. The analog of the ward attendant seemed to be the community worker. We knew very little about the procedures, practices and interventions used by community workers.

The initial efforts of the Committee to inform itself about these matters have been revealing and provocative. The community worker is a vital force influencing health and mental health delivery systems. In an attempt to offer some perspective by which the professional may perceive the role and function of the community worker, a number of issues crystallized in the course of the Committee's deliberations.

Are we abetting subtle forms of racism and/or elitism by rendering the most highly trained personnel relatively inaccessible to those patients with the most complex needs? This additional source of manpower (the community worker) has been used in some centers as just another way of offering inadequately trained and less skilled personnel to deliver services for that population or group with complex multifaceted problems.

In the absence of adequate mental health services, and

given the devastating effects of poverty, there are significant social and professional forces that support covert distancing maneuvers and avoidance techniques by interposing the community worker between the individual in need and the professional services to which he is entitled. Community workers should not be utilized to slight and deny those already neglected by currently operating mental health facilities.

The decision to use or not to use community workers must be based on a clear therapeutic rationale. Thus, it is essential to identify those individuals who are good candidates for intervention by the community worker, and those who would not benefit from the interventions of the community worker.

These issues are being actively considered in community health facilities, and although many aspects of them have been dealt with in foregoing sections of this report, further exploration and development are well warranted. The dynamic process involved in expanding an understanding of these issues requires active participation from a broad spectrum of health and psychiatric personnel, of necessity accompanied by inevitable confrontations of differing values, attitudes and orientations. In this final chapter of the report, we shall deal with some of these questions, mindful of the fact that many of the issues remain unresolved and unanswered in the report.

Workers' activities

The actual service delivered by the community worker is the crucial factor of community mental health practice that has received the least attention from other professional disciplines. The political and social nature of the community health worker movement has trained our focus on other crucial issues, thus diverting attention from the community worker-patient/client interaction.

The Committee's effort has been directed to a conceptualization of the human need system within which the community worker functions, and to the nature of the community worker's intervention with his client/patient. It is clear that the activities of the community worker are unique, and require greater attention to their nature and effectiveness.

Manpower potential

One of the major concerns for medicine in this decade is how to mobilize, prepare and utilize the most manpower potential available. It has been documented very clearly that the total number of medical and psychiatric personnel is not as great as that required to meet the tremendous need, nor do such personnel practice in the areas of greatest need. This situation has led to a widening separation of those patients most in need of service from the caregivers most able to deliver it.

The recently emerging interest in community health and community mental health highlights another aspect of this continuing concern. Community health centers, neighborhood health centers, outreach centers, and community mental health centers are all part of the attempt to make mental health services more accessible to those who need them, and acceptable to all patients, particularly those of moderate and low income, whether for primary, secondary or tertiary intervention. The reasons for this new approach are complex, but certainly are based on recognition of (1) the need to reach earlier than we do now those patients most in need, and in addition (2) the need to insure earlier case finding, maintain continuity of care, make services more readily accessible, and minimize the need for hospitalization.

Community workers have been recruited in large numbers to augment the manpower pool in the health professions. They are to be found especially in the low-income areas, poor neighborhoods, and localities settled by one or more minorities. The Committee has pointed out in preceding sections of this report their value in relation to patient-clients as helpers, educators, advocates and facilitators. In the Committee's collective view, they can be just as useful in non-poverty areas, particularly in bringing service to categories of individuals with special concerns such as the elderly, adolescents, and drug or alcohol abusers. The concept of the facilitator and helper acting also as advocate is a sound one and should not be restricted by any need among the professions to view their activities as helpful only to poor people.

The special usefulness of ethnic identification between helper and patient/client has been noted with reference to blacks and Spanish-speaking people. Such ethnic identification likewise facilitates the helping process when the helper can speak Yiddish in a Jewish, or Italian in an Italian, neighborhood. And it is of course true for as many subcultures as exist in our country. This is not to say that only a person having such an ethnic identification with a particular subculture can be helpful as a community worker, but rather to point out that the special attribute of ethnic identification can often be a vital component of the helping process.

Role definition

What are the limits and boundaries of the community workers' responsibility? Are they acting as agents of the physician, the social worker, or the nurse (who is then legally responsible for their therapeutic activities)? Similar questions can be asked about the role of all mental health disciplines.

Community workers consistently describe themselves as frontline personnel who function as a first line of operation whenever and wherever need dictates. Many examples have been cited in this report of their flexibility, their willingness to involve themselves in difficult therapeutic situations where the needs are not always readily apparent. In many situations they can act more quickly and decisively than a professional confronted with a similar circumstance because of their lesser need to unlearn patterns of behavior prescribed by the intervenor's role.

As a member of the more traditional psychiatric team, the community worker takes on a new role. A full description of this role, staking out its areas of expertise and competence, as well as its constraints and boundaries, awaits its unfolding development in this setting. Community workers are not necessarily certain that the full range of their potential usefulness has been explored. They enter their role as community worker with vastly differing experiences, levels of training, and orientations. It should not be at all surprising that their interests, skills, expectations and aspirations vary considerably.

The task of assisting in the exploration of the multiple functions and activities of the community worker will involve community workers themselves, and other health caregivers as well, to the extent that they interact with the community worker. Community workers cannot determine in isolation the full potential of their role. As a member of a team their role will shape itself to, and be modified by, the other team members. The value of the community worker's specific skills has already been pointed out earlier in this report, and it is these skills that must be meshed in with the total team effort.

Is there an active role for the community worker in the ongoing treatment process for a patient/client after the initial assessment of needs and the mobilization of institutional services in the patient/client's interests? What role can the community worker play in primary, secondary, and tertiary prevention? These two questions are being asked, and in part answered, at a number of community facilities. In many centers, community workers are assigned cases for supportive treatment, under the supervision of more skilled community workers and psychiatrists and other mental health professionals. Often they are the primary caretakers of a group of patient-clients, and thus in a position to make judgments and decisions that greatly influence the overall care of the patient/client.

As community workers evolve their sense of identity, they have begun to band together in increasingly more structured organizations to "professionalize" their roles, to discuss patient/client care issues, to form collective bargaining groups, and to unionize in their own best interests. This movement to form a group of "new professionals," as they are called in several cities, exerts a strong independent thrust and presents another challenge to medical psychiatric personnel.

Professional-nonprofessional struggles

The natural consequence of using community workers in medical-psychiatric-community mental health settings, and the slowly evolving sense of their role in these settings, forecast a series of inevitable confrontations between professionals and nonprofessionals. As already noted, community workers are not content with nonprofessional status, but are seeking to professionalize their status. This effort is particularly noticeable in a setting where professional status is equivalent to "first class" and nonprofessional status equivalent to "second class" or lower.

This kind of professionalizing by community workers elicits a variety of responses from individual nurses, social workers, psychologists and psychiatrists. Some view this striving as a healthy influence on a caretaking system that has become rigid, whose participants are unwilling to consider new treatment possibilities or new ways of intervening in the interests of good patient care. Others view the utilization of community workers, and the inevitable issues resulting from their utilization, as an unnecessary burden detracting from the delivery of quality care. To this latter group, efforts to legitimate and professionalize the community worker's role constitute an incursion upon territory traditionally occupied by themselves and other professionally educated and trained categories.

The resulting struggles between professionals and nonprofessionals are so severe in some medical-psychiatric-community mental health settings that patient/client care does suffer tremendously. In fact, these struggles attain such magnitude that patient-clients are lost in the battle. In the opinion of Committee members, this is the worst possible outcome of the inevitable confrontations between the two groups. Concern for patient/client care dictates that the issues, so difficult to resolve, which underlie these struggles must be worked through without delay wherever they evidence themselves. Some of the more concrete among their number may be posed as questions:

—LEADERSHIP: When there is a team approach to patient/client care, the community worker may direct, organize and coordinate the team's activities. *How does this leadership role, when played by the community worker, threaten the authority of the physician, nurse, or social worker?*

—FINANCIAL REWARDS: *If community workers are leaders, should they not be paid at a level commensurate with that of a leader? What are the implications of attempting to redistribute or reallocate the limited financial resources available?*

—COMMUNITY COMMITMENT: Community workers often lambaste professionals living outside the area to be served, who have different cultural backgrounds from those they serve, as not truly committed to the uncompromising delivery of quality care. The values and orientations of such professionals are continually being tested by community workers, as is their sensitivity to the factors of race, culture and poverty. *If the professional is never perceived as sensitive to racial, cultural, and economic factors, will he be able to continue to work in this setting? How can his understanding of his patients and their problems be enhanced and/or made manifest to patient/client and community worker?*

—PROFESSIONALIZATION: *If community workers are successful in their attempts to professionalize, won't they, too, become as rigid, inflexible, insensitive and bureaucratized as the professionals they now attack? What safeguards must be instituted to avoid this pitfall?*

Training of and by the community worker

Section 4 raises important questions about the specifics of community worker training. The Committee considers it important to reiterate and expand upon these questions here, and to point also to another major area for consideration—the training of professionals by community workers.

In considering the training of community workers, it is important to emphasize that confusion exists about the meaning of the term *training,* because of the multiple definitions currently accorded this word. As used here, the term *training* covers two major (training) areas: (a) inservice training in technical skills required for the specific tasks to be performed by the community worker, and (b) educational efforts by the community worker leading to the acquisition of conceptual knowledge and expanded techniques.

Community health and mental health centers must be continually concerned with four aspects of community worker training:

1) Inservice training under clinical supervision that will be usefully related to the tasks to be performed. Such training must be continually monitored and evaluated if it is to meet the needs of the community workers for whom it is designed. There must be sufficient supervision and/or consultation available for community workers functioning as primary caretakers in regard to their handling of transference, countertransference, and other methods of intervention likely to occur in the provider relationship with the patient/client.

2) More formalized training and education, with a more academic thrust, that can also be used as a stepping stone to additional future training. Too often such training is offered as a thing in itself which from a career standpoint leads to a dead end, with no horizontal or vertical mobility in the adjunct job situation. Not all community workers desire horizontal or vertical mobility, and that is a laudable option which should be supported. On the other hand, alternatives that offer an opportunity for further growth or expansion in the job hierarchy are vital.

3) Educational accreditation, which must be closely tied in with increased opportunities for financial reward if it is to be encouraged. This is not to say that every training course satisfactorily completed should result in an incremental salary adjustment, but it certainly implies that tangible reward must be accorded an increased level of competence and ability, especially to those receiving the lowest financial remuneration on the therapeutic team.

4) "Categorizing" the community worker. Categorization of the community worker reflects a grouping process intended to distinguish among them on the basis of their skills, competence and ability before further training. It can also be used, however, to favor those with the greatest verbal facility who reflect acceptable qualities of the dominant culture and are therefore rewarded by their selection for being reasonable facsimiles of many professionals' concept of the "generalized other." This close patterning to the other mental health disciplines can lead to an elitism that precipitates intragroup rivalry and dissension—already a too dominant feature of current mental health practice.

One type of training not specifically considered in community health and mental health centers—*the training of professionals by community workers*—is a relatively new but important concern. In the course of their investigations, Committee members observed increasingly that the information and knowledge about patient-clients flowed in both directions, from the professional to the community worker and from the community worker to the professional. Obviously in such a situation each has something to learn from the other. Yet it seems easier for most of those concerned to visualize professionals teaching community workers than the reverse. In part, this contrast in attitude may be sharpened by the acceptance on the part of many professionals, without critical examination, of the belief that they have little or nothing to learn from community workers.

The Committee is of the opinion, on the basis of its study, that there is definite value in involving community workers as teachers of other mental health professionals. Some of the areas in which they would be most competent are precisely those in which other mental health personnel may be the least knowledgable:

1—Specific community values, needs and expectations.
2—The community milieu—how it functions, the interrelated dynamic forces that shape it, the balance of power within the community and how that will influence health center planning.
3—How to enhance the process of entry into the community; what to do to remain there; and when and how to disengage from it.
4—The pitfalls of home visiting; the points at which intervention may reinforce a negative therapeutic alliance; and the kinds of intervention that are likely to be perceived as unhelpful by community residents.
5—Specific cultural, religious, linguistic or racial mores within the community that must be observed and respected by any potential helper.
6—Influence of the professional training given to the community worker and how this training enhances or interferes with the community worker's effectiveness.

This listing is intended to provide points of departure, from which important concepts and ideas can be developed and disseminated by the community worker in the specific situation.

Problem areas for community workers

Early in its observations, Committee members became aware that community workers experience a number of difficulties besetting their helping role. The problems encountered are somewhat similar to those experienced by all therapeutic intervenors. Some of them are particularly characteristic for community workers. Chief among these problems, perhaps, was the issue of a subjectively determined response. The manner in which this problem manifested itself was clearly apparent.

A number of community workers reacted toward their patient/client in ways determined by the internal dynamics of the helper rather than of the patient/client. In some instances, the inability of the community worker to recognize his own limitations and his lack of a specific skill in dealing with a particular patient/client prevented him from making available quickly and efficiently the care most appropriate to his client's needs. This tendency to assume competence in areas where it cannot be assumed poses a problem for some workers, many of whom have not yet learned that it is a sign of strength rather than weakness to request advice, assistance, or relief.

A common problem of community workers is to overidentify with the patient/client, and thus fail to maintain an objective distance from the complex issues being presented. This lack of "distance" makes for personalization of the issues and overidentification with the patient/client's situation. Many clear-cut decisions and options are easily overlooked once this process takes place. Another result of this overidentification is the sense of impotence and frustration felt by the helper when solutions to his patient/client's problems are not immediately at hand.

Confidentiality—always a problem for helpers at any level—is particularly a problem for community workers, who often know a patient/client or his family personally and live in the same immediate vicinity. It becomes an intricate matter to decide what to disclose and what limits to set on discussions about a patient/client. This is an area calling for constant attention and the inculcation of a specific orientation which recognizes the importance of sharing information as protected by certain restraints.

In a previous section on training, the Committee discusses the professionalization of community workers with reference to the worker himself. In addition to the issues raised there, however, the patient/client must be considered, for there is always the need for the worker to communicate between the patient/client and various helping institutions, and to coordinate needs with services. As community workers become more qualified like other professionals, and as they tend to identify with the values and orientations of institutions rather than those of a community constituency, their credibility and value in a mediating role between patient/client and institution are reduced and undercut.

Thus they become entrapped in a kind of limbo wherein they are identified with the service institutions too strongly for their patient-clients to perceive them as allies, while from the institutions' point of view they no longer speak for the grass-roots community. In this situation, the community worker who has become too much like the other professionals on the therapeutic team has lost his primary value to the team by losing his unique perspective.

These and similar problems comprise the daily staple for some community workers and the health units in which they function. Their resolution must be constantly sought in order to insure delivery of quality patient/client care.

Legal responsibility for the community worker

Although briefly mentioned in a previous section of this report, the question of legal responsibility deserves closer attention. The overriding question is, simply, who is responsible for the activities of the community worker? In an era of increasing malpractice suits and greater monitoring of patient/client activities by all third-party carriers, accountability and the responsibility for therapeutic activities must be clearly delineated and documented. In some health and community agencies, another question arises: Can third-party carriers be billed for the services of community workers? Will they accept verifiable activities by community workers as part of their reimbursable service contract? Federal, state and local municipalities, as well as private third-party carriers, are not uniformly agreed on the answer.

Many professional health and mental health workers are

beginning also to ask whether they are responsible for the community workers they supervise when legal complications arise. Are such community workers *their* agents, and in this event do they function on the professional's state or local license? The possible requirement to accept assumption of legal responsibility along with the supervision of community workers is enough, in some instances, to cause the health center problems in finding suitable supervision for community worker activities.

Should the movement to professionalize community workers gain momentum, the issue of their independent licensing by a state licensing board will become an active one. Any attempt to obtain licensure will call for a documentation of training and experience which can be generally, as well as specifically, replicated. Monitoring and quality control procedures, combined with periodic review, would be incorporated as part of the licensing and sanctioning mechanism. It is much too early to speculate further on this possibility, but the matter deserves mention here as an eventual solution of the current question concerning legal responsibility.

Other areas of concern

Sex of the community worker. Earlier in this report the Committee noted that in the urban community health and mental health centers visited, there were more women than men employed as community workers. Members were curious about the greater utilization of women in this category. The reasons for it appear to involve an intersecting montage of disparate limiting factors:

- —*Salary range available for the job.* When salary is low and noncompetitive, it virtually eliminates as candidates men who may be heads of households and cannot or will not work for the offered wage.
- —*Availability of men for the job.* There are certainly a large number of men looking for work, but there seems to be a

predominance of women among those actually applying for this job.

—*Willingness of men to function in a category of relatively low status.* Men may be especially sensitive to this aspect of the job, which also has a large caregiving and caretaking component that may appear too maternal or demanding to some men.

It has been reported by some married female community workers that when they have been offered the option of vertical mobility as a result of their training and competence, they accept with reluctance. This personal upward climb, without an accompanying upward spiral in the husband's job, has led to severe marital tension. The husband often feels left behind in a competitive sense and expresses concern about the possible loss of his position as head of the household. He also fears that his wife is becoming "too smart," and that she will be less interested in him.

Community and institutional change. Community workers in some health and mental health programs have been the catalyst for institutional change. This catalytic function is often the result of active and dedicated consultation and confrontation within the institutional hierarchy. Another time-honored approach some community workers employ in the catalyzing effort is organizing the community to confront the institution. Furthermore, the role of the community worker as community organizer dedicated to institutional change is likely to expand in the future.

There are three objectives leading to institutional change most often discussed by community workers. The first is to make the institution more responsive to the unmet service needs of the community. The second is to heighten the awareness of individuals within the institution to the negative influence of institutional racism on the community. The third is to advocate the sharing of institutional power with the community, which would involve community representation in the decision-making processes that affect the delivery of services.

A pertinent question to be answered in this connection is, what is the role of a health or mental health center in assuming responsibility for widespread *community* change? Increasingly in recent years, community health facilities, because of their visibility and accessibility, have become the focus of community pressure to effect widespread community change—in areas far beyond the delivery of health care—for example, in housing, welfare and education. Community workers functioning within the health or mental health center have been instrumental in directing institutional attention to these legitimate community concerns. How prepared is the health facility for a role in community leadership? Is this an appropriate role for the health facility? Why or why not? Does the community health or mental health center have a moral obligation and responsibility to accept this difficult challenge? These questions are often a daily concern of most such centers.

CONCLUSION

This report has focused primarily on the community worker as one who responds to human needs, and on the patterns and principles of the worker's intervention. The Committee's interest in the organizational, training, supervisory, and institutional issues dealt with is pertinent to the extent that these issues directly influence the nature and quality of the worker's intervention.

The issues raised here are important ones, directly influencing as they do patterns of service delivery and staffing patterns for community health and mental health centers. It is the considered opinion of the Committee as a whole that to understand the dynamic process occurring in health and mental health centers in relation to these issues is to be prepared for the crucial tasks ahead.

APPENDIX

TABLE 1—LISTING
Community Service Centers Visited by the Committee on Therapeutic Care

Area B Community Health Center	Washington, D.C.
Arlington Mental Health Center	Arlington, Va.
Baltimore Psychiatric Day Center	Baltimore, Md.
Brotherhood of Man	Towson, Md.
Model Cities Family Life Center (Mary E. Mahoney Center)	Boston, Mass.
OEO-sponsored Neighborhood Health Center	Philadelphia, Pa.
Orange-Person County Comprehensive Community Mental Health Center	Chapel Hill, N. C.
Rockville Health Center-Community Mental Health Field Service	Rockville, Md.
St. Elizabeths Hospital	Washington, D.C.
Sheppard and Enoch Pratt Hospital Crisis and Evaluation Clinic	Towson, Md.
South End Community Health Center	Boston, Mass.
South End Neighborhood Action Program (SNAP)	Boston, Mass.
West Philadelphia Community Mental Health Consortium	Philadelphia, Pa.

TABLE 2 — OUTLINE

Criteria of Acceptability for Study Data of Report

I—*Definition of agencies to be considered:* They will generally be viewed as "outreach" programs. Some partial hospital programs have affiliated closely with an institution and are borderline in the sense that they are so closely tied to the institution that there is actually very little in the way of outreach. Nevertheless, such programs can still be considered within the scope of the interest.

In the other direction, there are programs that are so loosely associated to any kind of organized health activities that they may be on the borderline in the sense that they reach out too far. Nevertheless, such programs may be looked at to get the full spectrum.

In general, the types of programs to be studied are storefronts, outposts, walk-in programs, home visits, neighborhood health centers, drop-in centers, hot-line services, emergency service-crisis intervention clinics, and special services in such places as schools and courts.

II—*Items to be studied:*

1. *Description of the agency*—The auspices, the structure of the organization (chart), the origins, the financing, formally defined interrelationships with other agencies, consumer participation.
2. *Biography of the worker*—Age, sex, race, education, experience, marital status, children; whether he has lived in the community, whether he is living there now.
3. *Philosophy of the worker*—How he entered into his position; what his goals with clients are; how he defines his role, kinship with the area, or commitment to the area; any ideas he may have about what helps people; constraints that are imposed by the role definition; the supports or assistance available to him in terms of supervision, access to other helpers, and consultation.

III—*Cases to be studied:*

1. How was the initial contact made?
2. How does the client define his needs?
3. How does the worker define the client's needs?
4. What interventions were made?
5. What additional help was needed?
6. What follow-up has there been?

TABLE 3

Specific Titles within the Generic Title of Community Worker*

Art therapist	Indigenous therapist
Child care worker	Mental health aide
Community advocate	Mental health counselor
Community coordinator	Mental health rehabilitation worker
Community health aide	Mental health technician
Community mental health worker	Mental health worker
Community worker	Neighborhood subprofessional
Ex-addict counselor	Neighborhood worker
Ex-alcoholic counselor	New careerist
Ex-mental hospital patient counselor	New professional
Expediter	Nonprofessional
Health education aide	Outreach worker
Health services aide	Paraprofessional
Home health aide	Preprofessional
Human service aide	Psychiatric technician
Indigenous aide	Social work aide
Indigenous health aide	Sociotherapist
Indigenous nonprofessional	Subprofessional

* This listing is not to be considered all-inclusive.

TABLE 4

Grouping of Designations for the Community Worker, by Category

I AIDES

Community health aide
Health education aide
Health services aide
Home health aide
Human service aide
Indigenous aide
Indigenous health aide
Mental health aide
Social work aide

II WORKERS

Child care worker
Community mental health worker
Community worker
Mental health rehabilitation worker
Mental health worker
Neighborhood worker
Outreach worker

III PROFESSIONALS

Indigenous nonprofessional
Neighborhood subprofessional
New professional
Nonprofessional
Paraprofessional
Preprofessional
Subprofessional

IV COUNSELORS

Ex-addict counselor
Ex-alcoholic counselor
Ex-mental hospital patient counselor
Mental health counselor

V TECHNICIANS

Mental health technician
Psychiatric technician

VI THERAPISTS

Art therapist
Indigenous therapist
Sociotherapist

VII OTHER CATEGORIES

Community advocate
Community coordinator
Expediter
New careerist

TABLE 5

Selected Grouping of Community Worker Designations by Other Broad Variables*

Designation	*Commonality with Patient/Client*
GROUP I:	
Community mental health worker Community worker Indigenous health aide Indigenous worker Neighborhood worker Outreach worker	Birth, culture, life style, life experiences
GROUP II:	
Ex-addict counselor Ex-alcoholic counselor Ex-mental hospital patient counselor	Similar problem or affliction, hence similar life style, life experiences, and subculture
GROUP III:	
New careerist New professional Paraprofessional Preprofessional Subprofessional	Relatively untrained formally in theory and practice of health and mental health; lack of academic credentials (degrees) or degrees not in health or mental health programs

* Neither categories nor commonalities are intended to be all-inclusive and may be frequently observed in various combinations.

FOR FURTHER READING: A PARTIAL BIBLIOGRAPHY

1. T. Elaine Adamson. Critical Issues in the Use of Physician Associates and Assistants, *American Journal of Public Health* 61, 9 (Sept 1971).
2. American Psychiatric Association. White Paper Prepared by The Commission on Manpower (Washington, D. C.: APA, 1966).
3. H. Aronson & Betty Overall. Treatment Expectations of Patients in Two Social Classes, *Social Work* 11 (1966): 35-41.
4. M. Bard & B. Berkowitz. Training Police as Specialists in Family Crisis Intervention: A Community Psychology Action Program, *Community Mental Health Journal* 3 (1967): 315-317.
5. A. A. Bartholomew & M. F. Kelly. The Personal Emergency Advisory Service, *Mental Hygiene* 46 (1962): 382-392.
6. J. C. Beck, D. Kantor & V. A. Gelineau. Follow-up Study of Chronic Psychotic Patients "Treated" by College Case-Aide Volunteers, *American Journal of Psychiatry* 120 (1963): 269-271.
7. L. Bellak. "Community Psychiatry: The Third Psychiatric Revolution," in HANDBOOK OF COMMUNITY PSYCHIATRY AND COMMUNITY MENTAL HEALTH, L. Bellak, Ed. (New York: Grune & Stratton, 1964) pp 1-11.
8. W. I. Bennett. Students, Patients Share Halfway House, *Rehabilitation Record* 5 (1964): 21-23.
9. Martin L. Birnbaum & Chester H. Jones. Activities of the Social Work Aides, *Social Casework* 48, 10 (1967): 626-632.
10. G. Brager. "New Concepts and Patterns of Service: the Mobilization for Youth Experience," in MENTAL HEALTH OF THE POOR, F. Riessman, J. Cohen & A. Pearl, Eds. (New York: The Free Press, 1964) 412-421.
11. ———. The Indigenous Worker: A New Approach to the Social Work Technician, *Social Work* 10 (1965): 27-32.
12. N. Q. Brill & H. A. Storrow. Social Class and Psychiatric Treatment, *Archives of General Psychiatry* 3 (1960): 340-344.
13. A. C. Brown. Psychiatrists' Interest in Community Mental Health Centers, *Community Mental Health Journal* 2 (1965): 256-261.

14. B. S. Brown & T. Ishiyama. Some Reflections on the Role of the Student in the Mental Hospital, *Community Mental Health Journal* 4 (1968): 509-518.
15. R. N. Butler & Lillian G. Sulliman. Psychiatric Contact with the Community-Resident, Emotionally Disturbed Elderly, *Journal of Nervous & Mental Disease* 137 (1963): 180-186.
16. Gerald & R. B. Caplan. "Developments of Community Psychiatry Concepts in the United States," in COMPREHENSIVE TEXTBOOK OF PSYCHIATRY, A. N. Freedman & H. I. Kaplan, Eds. (Baltimore, Md.: Williams & Wilkins, 1967) 1499-1516.
17. R. R. Carkhuff & C. B. Truax. Lay Mental Health Counseling: The Effects of Lay Group Counseling, *Journal of Consulting Psychology* 29 (1965): 426-431.
18. Center for Youth and Community Studies. TRAINING FOR NEW CAREERS (Washington, D. C.: CYCS, Howard University, 1965).
19. Abraham A. Chaplain, John M. Price, Jr., Isadore Zuckerman & Jon Ek. The Role of Volunteers in Community Mental Health Programs, *Community Mental Health Journal* 2, 3 (1966): 255-258.
20. June J. Christmas. Group Methods in Training and Practice: Nonprofessional Mental Health Personnel in a Deprived Community, *American Journal of Orthopsychiatry* 36 (1966): 410-419.
21. ———. Sociopsychiatric Treatment of Disadvantaged Psychotic Adults, *American Journal of Orthopsychiatry* 37 (1967): 93-100.
22. ———. Sociopsychiatric Rehabilitation in a Black Urban Ghetto. I: Conflicts, Issues and Directions, *American Journal of Orthopsychiatry* 39 (1969): 651-661.
23. June J. Christmas, Hilda Wallace & J. Edwards. New Careers and New Mental Health Services: Fantasy or Future? *American Journal of Psychiatry* 126 (1970): 1480-1486.
24. D. N. Daniels, A. B. Zelman & J. H. Campbell. Community-Based Task Groups in Recovery of Mental Patients, *Archives of General Psychiatry* 15 (1967): 215-228.
25. Ida F. Davidoff, Agnes C. Lauga & Robert S. Walzer. The Mental Health Rehabilitation Worker: A New Member of the Psychiatric Team, *Community Mental Health Journal* 5, 1 (1969): 46-54.

26. W. H. Denham *et al.* THE NEIGHBORHOOD WORKER: A NEW RESOURCE FOR COMMUNITY CHANGE. Monograph on the training and utilization of neighborhood workers. (Washington, D. C.: Center for Youth & Community Studies, Howard University, 1967).
27. Louis I. Dublin. "Suicide Prevention," in ON THE NATURE OF SUICIDE. E. S. Schneidman, Ed. (San Francisco, Calif.: Jossey-Bass, 1969) pp 43-47.
28. C. Eisdorfer & S. E. Golann. Principles for the Training of "New Professionals" in Mental Health, *Community Mental Health Journal* 5 (1969): 349-357.
29. R. B. Ellsworth. NONPROFESSIONALS IN PSYCHIATRIC REHABILITATION (New York: Appleton-Century-Crofts, 1968).
30. H. E. Freeman & D. G. Simmons. THE MENTAL PATIENT COMES HOME (New York: John Wiley & Sons, 1963).
31. A. Gartner. DO PARAPROFESSIONALS IMPROVE HUMAN SERVICES: A FIRST CRITICAL APPRAISAL OF THE DATA (New York: New Careers Development Center, 1969).
32. Alan Gartner & Frank Riessman. "The Performance of Paraprofessionals in the Mental Health Field," in AMERICAN HANDBOOK OF PSYCHIATRY, Gerald Caplan, Ed. (New York: Basic Books, 1971).
33. G. Goodman. "Companionship as Therapy: The Use of Nonprofessional Talent," in NEW DIRECTIONS IN CLIENT-CENTERED PSYCHOTHERAPY, T. Tomlinson & J. Hart, Eds. (New York: Houghton-Mifflin, 1968).
34. Milton Greenblatt, Paul E. Emery & Bernard C. Glueck, Eds. POVERTY AND MENTAL HEALTH, Psychiatric Research Report #21 (Washington, D. C.: American Psychiatric Association, Jan 1967).
35. C. Grosser, W. E. Henry & J. G. Kelly, Eds. NONPROFESSIONALS IN THE HUMAN SERVICES (San Francisco: Jossey-Bass, Inc., 1969). See especially articles by Gertrude S. Goldberg and Robert Reiff; and the Foreword by J. H. Scheuer. See also E. Hallowitz. The Role of a Neighborhood Service Center in Community Mental Health, *American Journal of Orthopsychiatry* 38 (1968): 705-714.
36. E. Hallowitz & F. Riessman. The Role of the Indigenous Nonprofessional in a Community Mental Health Neighborhood

Service Center Program, *American Journal of Orthopsychiatry* 37 (1967): 766-778.

37. N. Hansell, Mary Wodarczyk & H. Visotsky. The Mental Health Expediter, *Archives of General Psychiatry* 18 (1968): 392-399.
38. Norma J. Hart, Marcia Kroll, D. Berkowitz & Judith Woolcock. Assessment of Demonstration Community Mental Health Program by Its Nonprofessional Workers, *Proceedings 76th Annual Convention American Psychological Association* 3 (1968): 713-714.
39. Sam M. Heilig, Normal L. Farberow, Robert E. Litman & Edwin S. Schneidman. The Role of Nonprofessional Volunteers in a Suicide Prevention Center, *Community Mental Health Journal* 4, 4 (1968): 287-295.
40. Charles L. Hulin & Milton R. Blood. Job Enlargement, Individual Differences and Worker Responses, *Psychological Bulletin* 69 (1968): 41-45.
41. G. F. Hunter & Harold Stern. The Training of Mental Health Workers, *International Journal of Group Psychotherapy* 18, 1 (1968): 104-105.
42. Lewis & Adrianne Kadushin. The Ex-addict as a Member of the Therapeutic Team, *Community Mental Health Journal* 5, 5 (1969): 386-393.
43. Harold I. Lief. Subprofessional Training in Mental Health, *Archives of General Psychiatry* 6, 15 (1966): 660-664.
44. Mary Lynch & Elmer A. Gardner. Some Issues Raised in the Training of Paraprofessional Personnel as Clinic Therapists, *American Journal of Psychiatry* 126, 10 (Apr 1970): 1473-1479.
45. Mary Lynch, Elmer A. Gardner & Stanton B. Felzer. The Role of Indigenous Personnel as Clinical Therapists, *Archives of General Psychiatry* 19, 4 (1968): 428-434.
46. Ellen P. Manser, Jeweldean Jones & Selma B. Ortof. An Overview of Project ENABLE, *Social Casework* 48, 10 (1967): 609-617.
47. A. Pearl & F. Riessman. NEW CAREERS FOR THE POOR (New York: The Free Press, 1965).
48. H. B. Peck, S. R. Kaplan & M. Roman. Prevention, Treatment, and Social Action: A Strategy of Intervention in a Disadvantaged Urban Area, *American Journal of Orthopsychiatry* 36 (1966): 57-60.

49. Avis Pointer. NEW CAREERS: ENTRY-LEVEL TRAINING FOR THE HUMAN SERVICE AIDE (Washington, D. C.: National Institute for New Careers, 1969).
50. Robert Reiff & Frank Riessman. THE INDIGENOUS NONPROFESSIONAL: A STRATEGY OF CHANGE IN COMMUNITY ACTION AND COMMUNITY MENTAL HEALTH PROGRAMS, Monograph No. 1 *Community Mental Health Journal* (1965).
51. Hilda Richards & Marionette Daniels. Innovative Treatment Roles and Approaches, *American Journal of Orthopsychiatry* 39 (1969): 662-676.
52. Lincoln Richardson. Health is a Community Affair, *Presbyterian Life* (Jan 15, 1972): 16-20.
53. Frank Riessman. Strategies and Suggestions for Training Nonprofessionals. *Community Mental Health Journal* 3, 2 (Summer 1967): 103-110.
54. Margaret J. Rioch. Changing Concepts in the Training of Therapists. *Journal of Consulting Psychology* 30 (1966): 290-292.
55. ________. "Pilot Projects in Training Mental Health Counselors," in EMERGENT APPROACHES TO MENTAL HEALTH PROBLEMS, E. L. Cowen, E. A. Gardner & M. Zax, Eds. (New York: Appleton-Century-Crofts, 1967) pp 110-127.
56. Margaret J. Rioch *et al.* NIMH Pilot Study in Training Mental Health Counselors, *American Journal of Orthopsychiatry* 33 (1963): 678-689.
57. Margaret J. Rioch, C. Elkes & A. A. Flint. NIMH PILOT PROJECT IN TRAINING MENTAL HEALTH COUNSELORS, Pub. No. 1254 (Washington, D.C.: USDHEW, PHS, 1965).
58. Sheldon K. Schiff. Community Accountability and Mental Health Services, *Mental Hygiene* 54, 2 (Apr 1970): 205-214.
59. ________. Training the Professional, *University of Chicago Magazine* 62, 4 (Jan-Feb 1970): 9-14.
60. Sheldon K. Schiff & Douglass T. Turner. The Woodlawn School Mental Health Training Program: A Community-Based University Graduate Course, *Journal of School Psychology* 9, 3 (1971): 292-302.
61. E. Fuller Torrey. The Case for the Indigenous Therapist, *Archives of General Psychiatry* 20, 3 (1969): 365-373.
62. Charles B. Truax. The Training of Nonprofessional Person-

nel in Therapeutic Interpersonal Relationships, *American Journal of Public Health* 57, 10 (Oct 1967): 1778-1791.

63. R. M. Vidaver. The Mental Health Technician: Maryland's Design for a New Health Career, *American Journal of Psychiatry* 125 (1969): 1013-1023.

64. Shirley Wigfall & Anna H. Mace. A Paraprofessional Speaks, *Sandoz Psychiatric Spectator* (an Ortho Summary) Vol 8, No. 4 (1972) abstract.

ACKNOWLEDGMENTS TO CONTRIBUTORS

The program of the Group for the Advancement of Psychiatry, a nonprofit, tax-exempt organization, is made possible largely through the voluntary contributions and efforts of its members. For their financial assistance during the past fiscal year in helping it to fulfill its aims, GAP is grateful to the following:

Sponsors

J. Aron Charitable Foundation
CIBA-GEIGY Corporation, Pharmaceuticals Division
The Division Fund
Maurice Falk Medical Fund
The Grove Foundation
The Holzheimer Fund
Ittleson Family Foundation
Merck, Sharp & Dohme Laboratories
The Olin Foundation
Pfizer Laboratories
The Phillips Foundation
Roche Laboratories
Rockefeller Brothers Fund
Sandoz Pharmaceuticals
Schering Corporation
The Murray L. Silberstein Fund
The Lucille Ellis Simon Foundation
The Norton Simon Foundation
The Smart Family Foundation
Smith, Kline & French Laboratories
E. R. Squibb & Sons
The Sunnen Foundation
van Ameringen Foundation, Inc.
Leo S. Weil Foundation
Lawrence Weinberg
Weyerhaeuser Foundation, Inc.
Wyeth Laboratories

Donors

Fannie & Arnold Askin Foundation
Orrin Stine
The Stone Foundation, Inc.

OTHER PUBLICATIONS OF INTEREST
GROUP FOR THE ADVANCEMENT OF PSYCHIATRY

No.	Title	Price
89	Misuse of Psychiatry in the Criminal Courts: Competency to Stand Trial	$3.00
87	From Diagnosis to Treatment: An Approach to Treatment Planning for the Emotionally Disturbed Child	4.00
85	The Welfare System and Mental Health ...	1.50
77	Toward Therapeutic Care: A Guide for Those Who Work with the Mentally Ill ..	3.50
76	The Case History Method in the Study of Family Process	4.00
S-12	The Right to Die: Decision and Decision Makers (a symposium)	3.50

Orders amounting to less than $5.00 must be accompanied by remittance. All prices are subject to change without notice.

GAP publications may be ordered on a subscription basis. The current subscription cycle comprising the Volume IX Series covers the period from July 1, 1974 to June 30, 1977. For further information, write the Publications Office (see below).

Bound volumes of GAP publications issued since 1947 are also available which include GAP titles no longer in print and no longer available in any other form. A bound index to these volumes (I through VII) has been published separately.

Please send your order and remittance to: Publications Office, Group for the Advancement of Psychiatry, 419 Park Avenue South, New York, New York 10016.

This publication was produced for the Group for the Advancement of Psychiatry by the Mental Health Materials Center, Inc., New York